# SAVING LIVES

## WHY THE MEDIA'S PORTRAYAL OF NURSES PUTS US ALL AT RISK

SANDY SUMMERS, RN, MSN, MPH
AND HARRY JACOBS SUMMERS

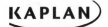

KAPLAN

PUBLISHING

New York

Lyrics from Aimee Mann's "Invisible Ink" used by permission of
Aimee Mann/SuperEgo Records.

© 2009 Sandy Summers and Harry Jacobs Summers

Published by Kaplan Publishing, a division of Kaplan, Inc.
1 Liberty Plaza, 24th Floor
New York, NY 10006

Library of Congress Cataloging-in-Publication Data

Summers, Sandy.
  Saving lives : why the media's portrayal of nurses puts healthcare at risk /
Sandy Summers and Harry Summers.
     p. ; cm.
Includes bibliographical references.
ISBN 978-1-4277-9845-9
1. Nurses in mass media. 2. Nursing--Public opinion. I. Summers, Harry.
II. Title.
[DNLM: 1. Nursing--standards. 2. Mass Media. 3. Nurse's Role.
WY 16 S956s 2009]
RT82.S886 2009
610.73--dc22
                                        2008048776

Printed in the United States of America

10 9 8 7 6 5 4 3 2 1

ISBN-13: 978-1-4277-9845-9

Kaplan Publishing books are available at special quantity discounts to use for sales promotions, employee premiums, or educational purposes. Please email our Special Sales Department to order or for more information at kaplanpublishing@kaplan.com, or write to Kaplan Publishing, 1 Liberty Plaza, 24th Floor, New York, NY 10006.

*For our children Cole and Simone*

*And their future nurses*

There comes a time when you swim or sink
So I jumped in the drink
'Cause I couldn't make myself clear
Maybe I wrote in invisible ink
Oh I've tried to think
How I could've made it appear.

But another illustration is wasted
'Cause the results are the same
I feel like a ghost
Who's trying to move your hands
Over some Ouija board
In the hopes I can spell out my name.

What some take for magic at first glance
Is just sleight of hand
Depending on what you believe
Something gets lost when you translate
It's hard to keep straight
Perspective is everything.

— Aimee Mann
from "Invisible Ink"
*Lost in Space* (2002)

# CONTENTS

# INTRODUCTION

NURSES SAVE LIVES EVERY DAY. But the media usually ignores their vital role in health care.

In 2005 U.S. Army Sergeant Tony Wood was riding in a Humvee in Iraq. A roadside bomb exploded. Metal tore into Wood's internal organs. A month later he woke up at Walter Reed Army Medical Center in Washington, DC. Wood first saw his wife—and asked what she was doing in Iraq. Wood's story appeared in an August 2008 *New York Times* article by Lizette Alvarez about traumatic brain injuries in combat veterans. Once Woods arrived at a hospital, expert nurses led the 24/7 effort that helped him survive, as they do with any patient whose injuries are so severe. But here is how Alvarez summed up that effort: "Doctors patched up most of his physical wounds over five months."

In a similar incident, a roadside bomb blew up near a Humvee in which U.S. Army Sergeant Nick Paupore was riding in Kirkuk City. Paupore lost his leg and an enormous amount of blood, but he too survived. In March 2008 the CNN website posted a story by Saundra Young about a Walter Reed neurologist's use of a promising new mirror therapy to help amputees like Paupore cope with phantom limb pain. Once again, nurses no doubt provided the great majority of the care that helped Paupore survive. But in describing the care Paupore received in Germany on his way to Walter Reed, the article reported simply that "doctors fought to save his life."

Meanwhile, starting in 2004, a new wave of television hospital dramas became popular around the world. On ABC's *Grey's Anatomy*, ten elite surgeon characters agonize adorably about love 'n' stuff and in their spare moments handle every meaningful aspect of patient care. On Fox's *House*, a witty, misanthropic genius leads a team of hospital physicians in diagnosing mysterious diseases, work which the show seems to equate with restoring patients to health. Once again, the show's physicians provide all important care.

When nurses do appear on these Hollywood shows, it is to mutely absorb physician commands, to move things, to serve as disposable romantic foils. The nurses are dramatic mirrors, reflecting light back on the beautiful physicians. And those physicians repeatedly mock nursing, making clear that they see it as a job for pathetic losers.

In this anxious post-9/11 world, we have found our heroes — and they aren't nurses. Sadly, the media often ignores nurses' real contributions to health. Instead, it presents nurses as low-skilled handmaidens, sex objects, or angels. In countless media products, only "doctors" receive credit for care that is actually provided by a team of nurses and other skilled health professionals. The media takes these popular misconceptions and strongly reinforces them.

Who cares?

You should. In reality, nurses are science professionals who save lives and improve patient outcomes every day. They monitor patients 24/7, provide high-tech treatments, advocate for patients, and teach them how to live with their conditions. But since the late 1990s, the world has suffered from a deadly shortage of nurses — the worst in modern history. A key element underlying many of the immediate causes of the shortage is poor public understanding of what nurses really do. That ignorance undermines nurses' claims to adequate staffing, nursing faculty, and other resources in our era of ruthless cost cutting.

*Saving Lives* explores what the public is told about the nurses who are fighting to save your life. We focus on the most universal source of public information: the media. We wrote the book to expand upon our work for the Center for Nursing Advocacy, a nonprofit organization dedicated to improving public understanding of nursing. Sandy and other graduate nursing students at Johns Hopkins founded the Center in 2001. Sandy had practiced nursing for fifteen years in emergency and critical care units at leading trauma centers in Washington, DC, San Francisco, and New Orleans. Sandy's husband Harry, a lawyer and media junkie, agreed to help the Center stir things up. Many nurses, nurse educators, and advocates rely on us to monitor and analyze what the media is doing, to advocate for more accurate portrayals of nursing, and to act as a resource for media creators with an interest in what nurses really do. We often use an approach we have called "entertainment advocacy," which aims to stimulate thinking in some of the same ways the media itself does, including irreverent and satirical elements.

Our advocacy has had a real impact on media creators. We have persuaded major corporations to reconsider advertising campaigns that relied on nursing stereotypes, such as a global Skechers campaign featuring Christina Aguilera as a "naughty nurse." We have helped companies rework ad campaigns to avoid nursing stereotypes. We persuaded the U.S. government to revise the name of an annual minority health care campaign to one that would not exclude the nurses who actually provide much of that care. News stories about our advocacy have appeared on major television networks and in print sources from the *Los Angeles Times* to the *Times of India*. And even Hollywood has reacted, grudgingly, to our analysis of its poor portrayal of nursing. We interact with producers, and some of them have been receptive to our concerns and advice, though far more needs to be done.

Of course, we also create controversy. Some people, including some nurses, cannot accept criticism of their favorite media products or challenges to the status quo generally. That criticism seems especially unwelcome when it comes from females in a traditionally female profession. Nurses are supposed to serve in silence! Nursing is about hearts and bedpans, not aggressive public advocacy, so shut up! Rock star Jack White accused us of "metaphorical ignorance" when we pointed out that one of his songs used nursing as a lazy metaphor for unskilled romantic care. Other critics deny that the popular media could affect the real world ("It's just a television show. Get over it!"). This attitude persists despite research to the contrary. It happens even though other fields (like education, politics, and advertising) rely on the same basic idea: what we see affects what we think and what we do. Still other critics insist that nursing can be helped only in some particular way other than what we do: therefore, we must stop what we're doing.

Because the global media has a keen interest in the many life-and-death issues in health care, the media that relates to nursing is vast. So this book is not comprehensive. It presents some basic ideas and notable recent examples. For in-depth treatment of the items discussed in this book, please consult the Center for Nursing Advocacy's website (www.nursingadvocacy.org) and materials cited there.

Here is a short summary of what you will find in *Saving Lives*. As we explain in chapter 1, nursing is a distinct scientific field and an autonomous profession. Nurses follow a holistic practice model that emphasizes preventative care and overall well-being. Virtually all U.S. nurses are now educated at colleges by nursing scholars. Nurses report to senior nurses, not physicians. Nurses practice in high-tech urban trauma centers and in vital health programs for poor mothers in bayou swamps. They work in leading research centers and in disaster zones. Nurses manage patient conditions, prevent deadly errors, teach and advocate for patients, and work for better health systems. But patients die when nurses are understaffed or underempowered, or when "nursing care" is assigned to those who are not nurses, in order to cut costs. The current nursing shortage kills thousands, if not millions, of people every year.

Chapter 2 shows how the media affects nursing. At times, the media offers an insightful look at what nurses really do. But usually nurses are portrayed as just the peripheral servants of heroic physicians. In 2008, thirty-nine out of forty-three major characters on the top five U.S. health-related prime-time television shows just "happened" to be physicians. The shows often present nursing as a job in a sad time warp. As Meredith Grey snapped at a male colleague in a 2005 *Grey's Anatomy* episode: "Did you just call me a *nurse*?!" Key factors in Hollywood's nursing problem include entrenched stereotypes, insufficient support from physicians, and nursing's own overall failure to represent itself well. Research shows that even entertainment television affects popular attitudes about health care generally and nursing specifically. Poor understanding leads to a lack of resources for nursing practice, education, and research, which in turn leads to worse patient outcomes, including death.

The media often portrays nursing with a mix of toxic female stereotypes. As we discuss in chapter 3, most media portrayals fail to convey that nurses are college-educated professionals who save lives. A few media items, particularly in the print press, have conveyed something of advanced nursing skills. Occasionally, this has even happened on NBC's *ER*! The most influential media, however, regularly sends the message that physicians are the sole masters of health knowledge and the only important staff in hospitals, even though hospitals exist mainly to provide nursing care. Contempt for nursing remains common. In a 2005 *House* episode, the godlike lead physician joked that picking up fallen patients was why he had "invented" nurses, calling out for one: "Cleanup on aisle three!" On Hollywood television shows, physician characters often do exciting things in which nurses would actually take the lead, like defibrillation, triage, and psychosocial care. Many news accounts assign credit for nurses' work to physicians, "hospitals," or machines. Other media ignores nursing, even when it actually plays a central role in the relevant topic, such as preventing hospital errors or responding to mass casualty events. Nurses are rarely recognized as health experts or important scholars. Of course, nurses may get credit for an isolated save outside their usual workplaces, which is news because it's a shock (Nurse passerby saves life?! Dog dials 9-1-1?!). Other items suggest that any helpful person or piece of health care technology is a "nurse." But "baby nurses" are no more nurses than they are babies.

Chapter 4 explores the prevailing media view of nurses as the faceless crew of a health care ship captained by charismatic physicians. Contrary to this view, nursing is an autonomous profession. Nurses train and manage themselves. They have independent legal duties to patients, and a unique scope of practice, including special expertise in areas like pain management and lactation research and practice. Hundreds of thousands have at least a master's degree in nursing. Occasionally media products have given some sense of nursing autonomy. These include infrequent news media items about nursing leaders or pioneering nursing research, and a few fictional portrayals, like the formidable Belize character in HBO's 2003 *Angels in America*. But the most influential entertainment media presents nurses as peripheral physician handmaidens. Every major Hollywood hospital show does so regularly, including *House, Grey's Anatomy*, and the NBC/

ABC sitcom *Scrubs*. The paradigmatic nurse-physician interaction is a physician "order" followed by a meek nurse's "Yes, doctor!"

The media often presents nurses as half-dressed bimbos. In chapter 5 we examine the staggering global prevalence of the "naughty nurse" image. It appears in television shows, music videos, sexually oriented products, and even the news media. In 2007, on *LIVE with Regis and Kelly*, Kelly Ripa promised to be a "sponge bath nurse" in her "little nursey costume" for co-host Regis Philbin, who was undergoing heart bypass surgery. Major corporations have used the naughty nurse to sell alcohol, razor blades, cosmetics, shoes, and even milk. The naughty image encompasses more subtle messages that nurses are mainly about the romantic pursuit of men, particularly physicians. Of course, the creators of naughty nurse imagery are "just joking"! But such social contempt discourages practicing and potential nurses, undermines nurses' claims to adequate resources, and encourages workplace sexual abuse — a major problem for real nurses.

Not surprisingly, nursing remains more than 90 percent female. Yet as we explain in chapter 6, media created by "feminists" has been hostile to nursing. Every major Hollywood hospital show of recent years has sent the message that nursing is not good enough for smart modern women. Films like the 2006 *Akeelah and the Bee* have celebrated the idea that promising girls, unlike their bitter mothers, do not have to settle for nursing. This same media is surprisingly open to the idea of men in nursing. But Hollywood's male nurse characters have at times served as vehicles for "feminist" role reversal. On ABC's *Private Practice,* cute nurse Dell is a clinic *receptionist* with virtually no health knowledge. Too much of the media defines success in terms of the power available in traditionally male jobs like medicine.

The media commonly presents nurses as angels of mercy or loving mothers, as we explain in chapter 7. Even many nurses and their supporters embrace the angel image. Johnson & Johnson's Campaign for Nursing's Future, which aims to address the nursing shortage, has run gooey, soft-focus television ads about "the importance of a nurse's touch." Compassion and caring are important parts of nursing, but the extreme emphasis on "angel" qualities reinforces the sense that nursing is not about thinking or advanced skills. And it implies that nurses, as virtuous spiritual beings, need little education, clinical support, or workplace security. It's true that nursing was traditionally seen as a religious vocation. But today, angel imagery suggests that nursing is not a serious modern profession and deters nurses from advocating for themselves and their patients.

Chapter 8 shows that the media often views nurses who do exert authority as battle-axes. The classic manifestation is the sociopathic Nurse Ratched in *One Flew Over the Cuckoo's Nest*, but the battle-axe has recently reemerged in prime time as a vindictive bureaucrat enforcing oppressive, trivial hospital rules. The battle-axe image seems to be the opposite of both the angel and the naughty images. But it is yet another one-dimensional female extreme. So while today's society may be ambivalent about punishing women *generally* for exercising power, it's still cool to punish women for trying to be powerful *nurses*. Sure, modern women are allowed to be tough and independent — as long as they pursue a traditionally male career.

As we discuss in chapter 9, advanced practice registered nurses (APRNs) provide care that includes tasks traditionally done by physicians. APRNs combine the holistic nursing care model with additional practitioner training, offering a hybrid approach that is changing health care. Contrary to the claims of some physicians, research shows that APRN care is *at least as effective* as that of physicians. Hollywood has offered a few well-meaning portrayals of APRNs, but these tend either to suggest that APRNs are skilled assistants to physicians or to show disdain, as in the mocking 2007 references to "midwifs" on *Private Practice*. Some news stories have conveyed a good sense of actual APRN practice, but APRNs are usually ignored as health experts. Some press accounts have suggested that APRNs can treat only minor problems. And the news and advertising media constantly reinforce the idea that practitioner care is provided only by "doctors."

Chapter 10 explains what *everyone* — not just nurses — can do to improve understanding of nursing. We can all try to look closely at the roles nurses really play in the health care system. And we can all consider how messages are embedded in our language, for instance our use of "nurse" to refer to any untrained caregiver. The media can try to convey a sense of what nursing really is. The news media should consult nurses when they actually have the expertise it needs. Hollywood should include characters to reflect the nurses who actually play central roles in the compelling health care it has shown physicians providing. Hospital managers should promote nursing as they do medicine. Governments and foundations must recognize the value of nursing. And more physicians should learn about the skills nurses have, then use physicians' social power to communicate that reality to the public.

But as we argue in chapter 11, nurses themselves must play the leading role in improving their image. Nurses should recognize that they have the power — and the responsibility — to foster change in their profession. They can start by projecting a professional image in everyday interactions, from how they deal with patients to the way they dress (we suggest fewer cartoon characters on scrubs). Nurses must work to help the media create more accurate depictions and persuade the media to reconsider harmful existing portrayals. And nurses should consider creating their own media to explain nursing directly, from writing letters to the editor to producing new Hollywood programs.

Nurses are the critical front-line caregivers in health care. For millions of people worldwide, nurses are the difference between life and death, self-sufficiency and dependency, hope and despair. Yet a lack of true appreciation for nursing has contributed to a shortage that is one of our most urgent public health crises. Many nurses feel that they've written in invisible ink, that their hard work is not understood, and the result is a lack of resources. The shortage of nurses is overwhelming the world's health systems. It is no exaggeration to say that our future depends on a better understanding of nursing.

Changing the way the world thinks about nursing may require a superhuman effort. But as the philosopher Albert Camus once wrote, "tasks are called superhuman when humans take a long time to complete them, that is all. The first thing is not to despair."

We can do it — if you help.

# PART ONE

# Dangerous Ignorance: Why Our Understanding of Nursing Matters

CHAPTER I

# Who Are Nurses and Where Have They Gone?

O NE NIGHT OUR FRIEND Dan Lynch had a patient who had just undergone a mechanical replacement of the aortic valve — the exit valve of the heart. As a cardiac surgical ICU nurse at a major hospital in Florida, Dan was monitoring the patient's heart that night with an arterial blood pressure line, among other ways. The art line, as it's called, is a tube that runs from an artery in the patient's wrist to a monitor, which displays in waveforms how well the heart is pumping blood through the arteries. Dan noticed that about every fifteen minutes the patient's art line waveform became flat. That could indicate that the patient's heart had stopped. Or, less dramatically, it could indicate that the art line's interior catheter had simply become kinked or stuck next to the arterial wall. After some moments, the patient's waveform returned to normal.

During the episodes, the heart monitor continued to indicate that the heart was beating normally. But Dan also noted that when the art line waveform became flat, the patient's central venous pressure

3

(CVP) monitor simultaneously failed to fluctuate in the expected waveform. Because the patient was still on the ventilator and heavily sedated, Dan was not able to measure if his level of consciousness dropped during these episodes. But Dan could not find a pulse at these times. Clearly, when the waveforms went flat, blood was not being pumped from the heart.

Dan concluded that the new aortic valve was sticking closed during the episodes. He called the surgeon at home and woke him up. The surgeon said that he had "never heard of such a thing" and that the art line was probably positioned incorrectly. Dan confirmed that this was not the case, and noted that even if it were, it would not explain the lack of pulse and lack of CVP waveform. The surgeon, unconvinced, hung up the phone. The charge nurse would not back Dan up because she too had "never heard of such a thing."

Dan called persistently, over the course of hours, until the surgeon finally came in to prove Dan wrong. But Dan wasn't wrong. It turned out that one of the stitches holding the valve in place was periodically obstructing its opening and closing—a problem that, left unaddressed even for a short time, could have killed the patient. The surgeon removed the stitch and resewed it. The patient survived.

The surgeon did not thank Dan for saving the patient, but he did allow that it was "the craziest thing" he'd ever seen. As far as Dan knows, neither the patient nor his family ever learned what Dan had done to save his life.

NURSES SAVE LIVES every day by using advanced skills and fighting for patients. But few people know it or even know what nursing is: a distinct scientific field. Nurses promote health and prevent illness. They follow a holistic practice model emphasizing a wide-angle view of health, with a strong focus on preventative care.

Nurses confront some of the most exciting challenges in health care. Their work settings range from the high-tech of teaching hospital ICUs to chaotic urban level-one trauma centers, from major research centers to community projects, war zones, and humanitarian relief projects around the world.

Nurses teach and advocate for patients. Nurses monitor and manage patient conditions, prevent deadly errors, provide skilled emotional support, perform key procedures, and work for better health systems. But if nurses are understaffed or underempowered, or if they simply make an error under pressure, patients can die.

Nursing is an autonomous profession.[1] Hospital nurses work with physicians, but they are managed by senior nurses. Some nurses lead hospitals. Physicians as a class lack the training and experience nurses have, and therefore, they cannot do nursing work.

Nurses are educated at colleges by nursing scholars who conduct cutting-edge research. Hundreds of thousands of nurses have graduate degrees in nursing. An increasing number have doctorates in nursing science. Nurses take rigorous exams to secure the government licenses they need to practice. And once licensed, nurses are bound by their own legal and ethical practice codes.

In addition to using the physiological expertise Dan Lynch displayed, nurses save lives in other ways. In a 2004 *American Journal of Nursing* article titled "Two Cups: The Healing Power of Tea," Hanne Dina Bernstein described how she cared for an emaciated leukemia patient who had recently had a bone marrow transplant.

The patient was depressed, refusing soup, grimacing at his medication, and refusing a newspaper. Bernstein took a pot of tea and two cups to the patient's room and declared, "I would like to watch the news." The patient was "clearly taken aback." He closed his eyes. Bernstein turned on the news and sat down.

Some time later Bernstein noticed that her patient was watching the TV. She told him that she had brought an extra cup of tea. The patient said he might have half a cup. The next night the patient had two cups of tea and a piece of toast, "his first solid food in a month." The following night the patient told Bernstein about his family, who lived too far away to visit. The fourth night the patient got out of bed.

A few days later he left the hospital, able to recuperate closer to home. Months later, while Bernstein was shopping, a "booming voice" greeted her. It was the now vigorous patient. He gave the nurse a hug and introduced her to his wife: "This is Hanne. She saved my life with a cup of tea."

She did. The story may bring a tear to readers' eyes, but consider the depth and importance of what Bernstein did. She quickly saw that the patient was depressed, alone, not eating—all of which could spell decline in a frail, critically ill patient. Though Bernstein initially felt "defeated," she decided to politely barge into her patient's life. At first the patient did not seem interested, but through her presence and the television, Bernstein reminded him of his connection to other humans. At the same time, she started him on the path to physical recovery with a cup of tea. She followed up in the ensuing days. The patient started eating and gaining strength. Of course almost anyone could physically do these things. But what average person would insist on "watching the news" in the room of a tired and depressed postoperative cancer patient?

But when nurses make mistakes, patients can die. Nurses have so many complex judgment calls to make—calls like Dan Lynch made with his heart patient or Bernstein with her leukemia patient—that it is easy to miss something, especially when a nurse is responsible for too many patients.

In 2006 veteran Wisconsin obstetrics nurse Julie Thao mistakenly gave a pregnant patient an epidural anesthetic into her IV, thinking the drug was penicillin prescribed for a strep infection. The anesthetic stopped the mother's heart and she died. (Her son was delivered alive by cesarean section.) Fatigue from excessive overtime and medication packaging problems may have contributed to the error. Thao, who expressed great remorse, later started a support group for nurses involved in serious errors. The case received national attention because Wisconsin for a time unwisely pursued a felony neglect charge against Thao.

Such high-profile cases are rare. In general, nurses operate under the radar, making health care function if they can. There are an estimated 12 million registered nurses worldwide. In the United States, there are about 3 million registered nurses. By comparison, there are about 700,000 physicians, a ratio of about four nurses to one physician. Nurses in the United States must have at least an associate's degree in nursing, which now requires about three years of rigorous college science work. About a million U.S. nurses have bachelor of science in nursing degrees. More than 375,000 hold at least a master's degree and 40,000 hold doctoral degrees. In the United States there are about 240,000 advanced practice nurses.[2] These nurses play leadership roles in clinical nursing and assume some duties traditionally performed by physicians, as nurse anesthetists do. Roughly 6 percent of U.S. nurses are men.

What exactly do all these nurses do?

- Nurses catch and halt life-threatening infections.
- Nurses coordinate the care provided by other health professionals, including physicians, social workers, and physical therapists.

- Nurses try to protect patients from inferior care, and some nurses risk their careers to blow the whistle on incompetence.[3]

- Nurses found and run new health systems for underserved communities, providing care to patients confronting obesity, prenatal difficulties, violence, and substance abuse.

- ICU nurses diagnose patients' wide-complex tachycardia, call a code, and defibrillate — saving the patients' lives.

- Emergency department nurses triage patients based on their own expert evaluation of who needs care first.

- Military nurses, as commissioned officers, manage complex military care operations around the world.

- Nurses provide much, if not most, of the health care given by aid groups like Doctors Without Borders.[4]

- Nurses manage violent, intoxicated patients alone until security gets there — *if* security gets there — and so nurses are most at risk for assault in a hospital setting.

- Nurses are the caregivers most likely to be present when patients are screaming, crying, laughing, or dying.

Real nursing is exciting. That's why major hospital shows on television, like *House* and *Grey's Anatomy*, spend so much time showing work that real nurses do. Sadly, they show physician characters doing it. But more on that later.

## A FEW NOTES ON NURSING HISTORY

The origins of nursing depend on what you think nursing is. Is it skilled professional health care or just any care? Family members have always cared for the sick. But calling that care "nursing" suggests that anyone is qualified to be a nurse.

Even in ancient times, groups of people cared for those who could not care for themselves. In the third century BCE, a school for male caregivers was established in India. Its practitioners focused on moral purity and skill, especially in cleaning beds. In the third century CE, the Parabolani order in Greece began caring for plague victims. The name Parabolani referred, aptly, to those who took a risk.

The roots of modern nursing are in religious and military settings. In the Middle Ages, European religious orders began to establish groups of trained caregivers. Saint Benedict founded such an order around 500 CE. Christian deacons and deaconesses did "the work of God" by caring for the sick. In the sixteenth century the Italian priest Saint Camillus worked to improve care in facilities for the ill and in the wider community. He developed the first ambulance and invented the sign of the red cross to represent care for the sick. In the seventeenth century, Saints Vincent de Paul and Louise de Marillac established the Sisters of Charity in France to provide health care to the poor. The Sisters did their nursing in patients' homes, on battlefields, and in their own facilities.

But by the nineteenth century, basic care was often provided by less religious individuals. In Europe a "nurse" was commonly thought of as a drunken woman of uncertain morality, such as Sairey Gamp in Charles Dickens's satirical 1844 novel *Martin Chuzzlewit*. In a sense, modern nursing has been caught between the "angel" and the "naughty" image from the beginning.

By the mid-nineteenth century, reformers in Europe and the United States sought to improve the horrific conditions the sick endured, in part by developing a cadre of dedicated female caregivers: nurses. In Bernice Buresh and Suzanne Gordon's influential

*From Silence to Voice* (2nd ed. 2006), and in Gordon's equally influential *Nursing Against the Odds* (2005), the authors show that when these reformers professionalized nursing, they sought to establish a respectable job for women outside the home.[5] They had to steer clear of the Gamp image, to enable the nurses to provide intimate care to strangers. The authors, relying in part on the work of nursing scholar Sioban Nelson, show that the reformers used a moral or "virtue" script—first Christian, later civic. Here are more roots of nursing's "angel" image. The reformers also assured male physicians that the female nurses would not challenge their authority over care or their scope of practice. We start to see the roots of nursing's "handmaiden" image.

The best-known of the reformers was Florence Nightingale, the fierce, brilliant British nurse. Nightingale's wealthy parents initially refused to let her become a nurse, but she managed to receive some hospital training, and in 1854, during the Crimean War, she led a group of nurses in providing care to wounded British soldiers near Constantinople. She soon became revered for her tireless efforts to improve conditions. Back in England, Nightingale tried to reform hospital conditions, military and civil, particularly in the area of sanitation. In 1860 she established the hospital-based Nightingale Training School for Nurses and published *Notes on Nursing*, which presented nursing as a distinct scientific profession. It is arguably the most influential book ever published about nursing. Nightingale's *Nursing Notes*, the first nursing journal, appeared in 1887. Nightingale also pioneered reforms in care delivery structures and the use of health statistics. Her work had a profound effect on health worldwide. Her nickname—the "Lady with the Lamp"—does not do justice to her accomplishments, though it does at least suggest her focus on close 24/7 observation.

Other nineteenth century figures also played key roles in the development of nursing, though not all had nursing training. In the middle decades of the century, Dorothea Dix worked to reform U.S. institutions caring for the mentally ill. Clara Barton organized and provided care to soldiers on the battlefields of the Civil War and later founded and led the American Red Cross. She was known as the "Angel of the Battlefield" ("Visionary Disaster Relief Leader" must not have caught on). Linda Richards was the first nurse to graduate from a U.S. nurse training school, at Boston's New England Hospital for Women and Children, in 1872. Richards later established several nurse training schools, including the first in Japan. In 1893 nurse Lillian Wald established New York's Henry Street Settlement, the first visiting nurse institution in the United States. Wald effectively created public health nursing and influenced care across the globe.

Though many very early caregivers were male, modern nursing has struggled from the beginning with its gender imbalance. Some men were considered to be acting as nurses during the American Civil War — most famously the poet Walt Whitman — but men were prevented from serving as U.S. military nurses or joining some nursing professional associations until well into the twentieth century.[6]

In the last century, nations began to license nurses, nursing education gradually moved from hospitals to universities, and nursing journals began to flourish. The University of Minnesota granted the first bachelor's degree in nursing in 1909. Yale established the first autonomous school of nursing in 1923. New York University established the first PhD program in nursing in 1934.

Meanwhile nurses were improving care in ways that cut against the grain of accepted practice. In the early part of the last century, Mary Breckinridge established the Frontier Nursing Service (FNS) in Kentucky, effectively founding American nurse-midwifery. The

FNS has saved the lives of many mothers and children, and it has served as a global model for rural health care delivery.[7]

In the 1960s New York nursing leader and theorist Lydia Hall established an influential nurse-centered rehabilitation hospital, the Loeb Center, where registered nurses provided all hands-on care. Physicians and other staff played only minor roles.[8]

As understanding and technology advanced, nurses managed increasingly complex patient conditions and care technologies. In the 1960s nurses began training as advanced practitioners in fields that included tasks traditionally done by physicians, though the nurses employed their own holistic approach. These advanced practice nurses, most with at least master's degrees in nursing, now provide high-quality care in areas such as family practice, anesthesia, and midwifery. At the same time, graduate-prepared clinical nurse specialists began providing clinical leadership to bedside nurses. In 2004 Columbia established the first doctorate of nursing practice program to award more comprehensive clinical degrees to advanced practice nurses. Nurses have taken the lead in developing better end-of-life care,[9] reducing domestic violence,[10] and improving pain management.[11] Nurses have pioneered cutting-edge fields such as health informatics, which focuses on managing the increasingly complex body of information in patient care.[12] And sexual assault forensic nurses represent the state of the art in caring for victims and assembling court evidence.[13]

In recent years nursing leaders have improved public health worldwide through research and innovation. Korean Susie Kim has pioneered new psychiatric treatments and cost-effective mental health centers for the developing world.[14] Kenyan Elizabeth Ngugi has saved countless lives by changing how AIDS care is delivered and studied in ostracized communities.[15] University of Pennsylvania professor Loretta Sweet Jemmott, one of the world's leading experts in preventing HIV transmission to youth, has led efforts to improve the health of underserved urban communities.[16] Jemmott's Penn colleague, prominent scholar Linda Aiken, has published a series of groundbreaking studies linking better working conditions for nurses, including higher staffing levels, with better patient outcomes.[17] Tennessee nurse Carol Etherington has worked to secure the health and human rights of vulnerable populations worldwide, creating effective programs for survivors of natural disaster, war, and other abuses.[18] Johns Hopkins nursing professor Jackie Campbell is one of the world's leading experts in understanding and reducing domestic violence.[19] And nurses like Ruth Lubic have led the struggle to increase U.S. use of nurse midwife–centered childbirth care, which the rest of the developed world employs to achieve better outcomes at a lower cost.[20]

For nursing, the future should be wide open. Nurses are more expert and in some ways more empowered than ever, and their holistic approach to public health is sorely needed. But a perfect storm of economic and social factors now poses a threat to nurses and their patients that may be unparalleled in modern times: the global nursing shortage.

## THE NURSING SHORTAGE

Since the late 1990s, the world has experienced one of the longest and worst nursing shortages in modern history. The shortage has had a devastating effect on patient outcomes — literally killing thousands, if not millions, of people every year.

Too few nurses are practicing today, and tomorrow looks even worse. A July 2007 report by the American Hospital Association estimated that U.S. hospitals needed about 116,000 nurses simply to fill currently vacant positions.[21] In November 2007 the U.S. Department of Labor estimated that more than one million new and replacement nurses will be needed by 2016.[22] And a March 2008 report by nursing scholars estimated that the shortage of U.S. nurses could reach 500,000 by 2025.[23] Other developed nations are experiencing similar shortfalls. Meanwhile, as developing nations struggle to finance their meager health care systems, many of their best nurses are emigrating to developed nations eager for their skills.

Immediate causes of the shortage are numerous. Many nurses leave the bedside because of nurse short-staffing or poor working conditions.[24] The nursing workforce is rapidly aging, as too few new nurses are being educated. Inadequate resources are devoted to nursing education, and there is a shortage of qualified faculty. Women in many nations have come to enjoy a far greater range of career choices than in the past. For the most part, women in nursing have not made the gains in workplace empowerment that their counterparts in many other professions have made. At the same time, men are still not entering nursing in significant numbers. Many do not consider the field because they do not know that what nurses do matters. Abusive treatment from physicians also continues to drive nurses from the workforce,[25] especially where nurses' status is low.[26] And while these problems continue, the demand for nurses has grown because of rapidly aging populations in developed nations and the increasing complexity of health care and care technology.

Short-staffing, driven by the undervaluation of nursing, is central to the crisis. Several key books have explored this, among them *Safety in Numbers* (2008) by Suzanne Gordon, John Buchanan, and Tanya Bretherton; Gordon's *Nursing Against the Odds* (2005); and Dana Beth Weinberg's *Code Green: Money-Driven Hospitals and the Dismantling of Nursing* (2003).[27] Many nursing positions were actually cut in the 1990s due to managed care, which had curtailed insurance reimbursement, threatening many care facilities. Many hospitals implemented restructuring plans that drastically increased the workloads of registered nurses. Nurses, who remained underempowered, lacked the resources to resist these threats to their patients and themselves. Many tasks formerly performed by nurses — tasks that enabled nurses to perform critical nursing assessments — were now done by unlicensed assistive personnel or not done at all. This is why even high nurse vacancy rates do not fully convey the scope of denursification in hospitals today. Most hospitals need many more nurses than they are actually seeking.

These conditions drove away many nurses who could no longer face their growing burnout and the realization that they could not meet their professional responsibilities to their patients.[28] By 2004 roughly half a million U.S. registered nurses (about one-sixth of the national total) had chosen not to work in nursing.

In recent years many reports have described what short-staffing does to nurses and patients. In February 2004 *Newsweek* ran Michigan ED nurse Paul Duke's powerful "If ER Nurses Crash, Will Patients Follow?" Duke's column told how chronic short-staffing was leading him to ask "Did I kill anyone today?" In five years Duke's patient loads had increased from four or five up to ten or twelve. In that environment, he wrote, nurses are "tired and beaten down." Duke vowed to continue with the profession he loved despite feeling "steamrolled," but nurses in general cannot be expected to do so.[29]

In October 2003 *Reader's Digest* published an anonymous ICU nurse's powerful account of one shift in which she was expected to do the work of an EKG tech, nurses' aides, housekeepers, secretaries, and pharmacy delivery people. This overload kept her from giving patients critical medicines on time. Meanwhile, she was responsible for three ICU patients, though more than one or two is unsafe.

Her patients were an agitated man in restraints suffering alcohol withdrawal, a 300-pound woman with a serious blood infection, and a man with severe cerebral palsy suffering pneumonia and bedsores. The nurse constantly monitored the conditions of these patients and handled their difficult minute-to-minute needs. With the help of other nurses, she adjusted the overweight patient's position so she could breathe. The nurse stopped a dietary worker from giving the patient a meal that would have harmed her. For these key interventions, the nurse received abuse from the patient.

The nurse negotiated a change in a patient's medication to reduce his agitation and the likelihood of complications, despite resistance from junior physicians. The nurse coordinated relations among patients, their families, and other health workers, suffering abuse from family members for not being responsive enough. She also managed to provide skilled support and an Al-Anon referral to a patient's distraught mother. Miraculously, none of the nurse's patients appeared to suffer serious problems. But the nurse ended her piece by describing the physical pain the shift had caused her, noting, "How much longer I can work like this, I just don't know."[30]

These are not just isolated stories. A wealth of research links lower nurse staffing levels to nurse burnout and worse patient outcomes, including medication errors, serious complications, longer hospital stays, missed care from surveillance to feedings, and death.[31] Nursing scholar Linda Aiken and colleagues published an influential 2002 study in the *Journal of the American Medical Association* showing that postoperative patients whose nurse had eight patients had a 31 percent higher chance of dying than patients whose nurse had four patients.[32] In 2006 a study in *Health Affairs* showed that raising the number of registered nurses in hospitals would reduce millions of hospital days and save thousands of lives each year, at a relatively small or no cost.[33]

Globally, the nursing shortage is even more worrisome. In a 2004 report the International Council of Nurses (ICN) explained that key factors in the global shortage include the continuing threats of HIV/AIDS, nurse migration, and health sector reform and restructuring. The nurse-to-population ratio now varies greatly worldwide. The average ratio in Europe is ten times higher than that in Africa and South East Asia. Some nations, particularly in Central and South America, actually have more physicians than nurses. Bringing the nurse-to-population ratio seen in the most developed nations — roughly 1:100 — to the rest of the world would require 50 million additional nurses, for a total of five times the number of nurses we have now. Many nations also have a poor distribution of nurses, with few nurses in rural and remote areas. In explaining the shortage, the ICN report noted that "gender-based discrimination continues in many countries and cultures, with nursing being under-valued or downgraded as 'women's work.'"[34]

One of the most alarming global trends is the migration of developing world nurses (and physicians) to much better paying positions in developed nations with shortages. Notwithstanding the funds these workers send home, this trend has had a devastating impact on already overburdened health systems in poor nations. In a June 2007 article in *Health Services Research*, nursing migration expert Mireille Kingma explained that developed-world shortages had led to aggressive recruiting campaigns overseas. Yet Kingma argued that nurse migration was primarily a "symptom" of larger systemic problems that cause nurses to leave jobs, mainly poor salaries and working conditions. She noted that "no matter how attractive the pull factors of the destination country, little migration takes place without substantial push factors driving people away from the source country." Kingma concluded that "injecting migrant nurses into dysfunctional health systems — ones that are not capable of attracting and retaining domestic-educated staff — is not likely to meet the growing health needs of national populations."[35]

Legislative efforts to combat the shortage have not yet had a broad impact. Following the lead of the Australian state of Victoria, California has been the first U.S. state to impose mandatory minimum nurse staffing ratios, despite fierce opposition from the hospital and insurance industries, which argue that the ratios are impractical and may force hospitals to close. Other states, including Massachusetts and Florida, have considered legislation mandating specific minimum ratios.[36] The book *Safety in Numbers* argues strongly that mandatory minimum ratios, while not perfect, have proven a cost-effective way to improve working conditions, nurse retention, and patient outcomes in Victoria and California. The authors show that the horror scenarios predicted by hospitals have not materialized.

Recently legislation has been introduced in the U.S. Congress to address nurse staffing, including bills to set specific minimum nurse-patient ratios and to limit mandatory overtime. None of these bills has passed. The federal Nurse Reinvestment Act (2002) contains promising measures, including incentives to increase nursing faculty. But the Act has not received nearly enough funding to have a meaningful impact.[37]

Hospitals have responded to the shortage in various ways. Many have recruited nurses from overseas[38] and relied on nurse staffing agencies and travel agencies to supplement their staff.[39] Some hospitals have made efforts to improve working conditions, including staffing levels and scheduling policies. A relatively small number of hospitals, mostly in the United States, have earned Magnet status. The American Nurses' Credentialing Center awards Magnet status to hospitals that satisfy criteria designed to measure the strength and quality of their nursing, including nurses' participation in decision making, job satisfaction, low turnover, and appropriate grievance resolution. Some critics (including nursing unions) have argued that the program is inadequate since it lacks minimum nurse-to-patient ratios, that the nurse empowerment it offers is mostly illusory, and that hospitals have used it mainly as a promotional tool.[40]

Several media campaigns have aimed to address the nursing shortage. Perhaps the most prominent is Johnson & Johnson's ongoing Campaign for Nursing's Future, launched in 2002. The drug company has spent tens of millions of dollars on television ads, recruiting videos, a website, and scholarships. Some of these campaign efforts have been positive, but the television ads have often presented nursing in the same emotional, gendered ways in which the public already sees the profession, and so have done little to enhance real understanding.[41] Nurses for a Healthier Tomorrow (NHT), a coalition of health care groups, has tried to interest secondary school students in nursing through focus groups, a website, and other media activities. NHT's media efforts give specific examples of the life-saving value of nursing.[42] NHT has also worked to persuade nurses to become nurse educators.

In the last few years, U.S. interest in nursing has increased somewhat, probably helped by a weak economy and a growing awareness that nursing offers plentiful, diverse positions with the chance to better lives, along with starting pay that is good relative to the amount of formal training required. No doubt this awareness has been driven by extensive media coverage of the shortage and by the above media campaigns.

Unfortunately, simply training more nurses, like recruiting from other nations or regions, will do little to address many of the key underlying causes of the nursing shortage. Moreover, a critical shortage of nursing faculty has hampered efforts to educate more nurses, and nursing schools have turned away many qualified applicants.[43] A 2007 report by the National League for Nursing and the Carnegie Foundation found that nurse educators earn only three-fourths of what faculty in other academic disciplines earn and significantly less than other nurses with the same educational credentials, such as advanced practice nurses.[44] Nursing scholars get relatively little funding from the U.S. government. As of 2009, nursing research made up *less than half of one percent* of the budget for the National Institutes of Health.[45]

Reports in 2008 showed that the nursing shortage and nurse short-staffing remained critical problems throughout the world. The March 2008 study by nursing scholars made clear that the crisis in the United States is ongoing.[46] The picture elsewhere is often worse. On March 17, 2008, the Indian newspaper *The Hindu* ran a piece headlined "India Running Short of Two Million Nurses." The piece reported that nearly 20 percent of "experienced nurses" had left India for the United States or Europe.[47] That same day, Carol Natukunda's piece in Uganda's *New Vision* had discussed that nation's rampant nurse emigration. One official cited nurse-to-patient ratios of 1:1,000. The piece was entitled "Uganda: Where Did All the Nurses Go?"[48]

If the shortage continues as projected, it will have catastrophic effects. Already it severely hampers our ability to respond effectively to mass casualty events, since nurses would provide the great majority of the care those require. And in some nations, it is obstructing economic, social, and political development across the board. As the ICN report stressed, the nursing shortage is a public health crisis.

But as we argue in the rest of this book, a critical factor underlying the shortage is the huge gap between the *actual* nature and value of nursing, on the one hand, and what policy makers, career seekers, and the public at large *believe* about nursing on the other. Nursing has not received adequate resources because it continues to be seen as a peripheral, menial job for women with few other options. So it will not be enough to consider legislative reforms and to increase funding for nursing, as vital as these steps are. All the numbers measuring the shortage reflect what starts in our minds. The shortage cannot be resolved until public understanding improves. We must change how the world *thinks* about nursing.

## CHAPTER 2

# How Nursing's Image Affects Your Health

IN 2007 A FRIEND OF OURS got a phone call. Producers of a popular U.S. prime-time television hospital show that is seen around the world had found her name, presumably in a database of experts. The producers called for a script consult because our friend is a leading expert in a certain health field. Our friend gave the TV producers cutting-edge information to help them develop a plotline.

Our friend said that these Hollywood producers "were *super* surprised I was a nurse — and *super, super* surprised I had a PhD and was one of the leading researchers in the country on this issue." She also "took the opportunity to say quite a bit to them about nursing — both how nurses could be used in the story line and how their general approach to nursing could be substantively improved."

The result? The producers said the show's audience is "interested in doctors not nurses." They said there were no plans to have a nurse character with a significant role: "We have a stable cast and the focus of the show is on physicians." Do not attempt to adjust your television: the stereotypes are in control.

THIS IS A SELF-REINFORCING LOOP: Hollywood tells its audience that physicians' work is dramatic and important, and nursing is not, because that's what the audience expects. And the audience expects to see the stories of physicians rather than nurses in large part because that's what Hollywood presents as interesting and compelling TV. In fact, as we explained in chapter 1, real nursing work is highly dramatic[1] — which is why TV physicians spend so much time doing it. Even on the diagnosis-*über-alles* Fox drama *House*, physician characters spend a good deal of time doing what is really nursing work. However, it is presented as the work of physicians. The real physician role alone does not seem to be interesting enough to carry a TV drama.

The media has long been fascinated with health care, especially what goes on in hospitals. Countless health items appear daily in the various news media. And many of the most popular recent television series have been hospital shows.

Occasionally the media offers insight into what nurses really do. Examples include an excellent 2007 *Wall Street Journal* piece about editor John Blanton's experience as a new nurse, a 2007 series on the nursing shortage on WBUR (the Boston *National Public Radio* affiliate), and the 2003 HBO film *Angels in America*.

But most of the time nurses are presented as the peripheral and/or sexy servants to the heroic physicians who provide all important care — the care that saves or improves lives. Even the elite news media, like the *New York Times* and NPR, relentlessly equate "doctors" with all of health care. This is true even in areas like intensive care, in which nurses actually take the lead in keeping critical patients alive by constantly evaluating them and managing highly complex treatments. Research shows that nurses appear in 1 to 4 percent of health-related newspaper articles.[2] When nurses do appear, it's usually in pieces specifically about nursing's discontents — the nursing shortage, labor disputes, or extreme misconduct, like serial killing. It's relatively rare for the media to cover the life-saving work nurses do every day at their jobs or to consult nurses as the health care experts they really are.

The entertainment media is even more troubling. J. K. Rowling's vastly popular Harry Potter novels, published from 1997 to 2007, do include the very minor character Madam Pomfrey. This wizardry school nurse is single-handedly able to cure dragon bites, treat curses, and heal Harry after he falls fifty feet off a flying broom. But television remains in many ways the dominant global medium. In the 2007–2008 prime-time U.S. television season, the only new health drama was ABC's *Private Practice*, a spinoff of the network's ratings monster *Grey's Anatomy*. The show focuses on seven pretty, smart physicians practicing at a Los Angeles clinic. The last, and least, character is clinic receptionist Dell. Dell is a cute surfer boy — and a nurse studying midwifery, a field the show has mocked relentlessly. This character placed fourth in a May 2008 *TV Guide* poll of the "sexiest secretaries" on TV. Viewers failed to register that Dell's a graduate student with a bachelor of science degree in nursing.

Since 2005 *Grey's Anatomy* has shown its smart, attractive surgeon stars providing all significant care. Though appearances by nurses are few and far between, the lives of the nurses who do appear revolve around the physician characters. *Grey's* continues to vie with *House*, which began in 2004, to be the contemporary show most damaging to nursing. *House* also features a slew of smart, pretty physicians, led by the brilliant, acerbic lead character, Greg House. Again, these physicians provide all important bedside care. The show treats the few nurses who appear — to mutely absorb physician commands — with contempt. These two shows have regularly attracted 15 to 20 million U.S. viewers. And they are popular around the world.

Other shows are not much better. NBC's drama *ER* (1994–present) and the NBC/ABC sitcom *Scrubs* (2000–present) are overwhelmingly physician-centric. But each of those veteran shows does at least have one major nurse character who can think and talk. FX's edgy *Nip/Tuck* (2003–present), which follows the exploits of two ethically challenged plastic surgeons, has never had any. USA Network's *Dr. Steve-O* (2007–2008) featured *Jackass* veteran Steve-O in a reality show aimed at "de-wussifying wimps." That vital task involved macho stunts and the host's sidekick, naughty "nurse" Trishelle.

In 2008 the six health-oriented shows above (disregarding *Dr. Steve-O*) featured forty-one major physician characters and three major nurse characters. In early 2009 the premium cable network Showtime plans to introduce a half-hour "dark comedy" about a tough New York City emergency nurse, with the tentative title *Nurse Jackie*. We believe this will be the first major American prime-time show with a nurse character as the central focus since the early 1990s.

Research confirms that the media plays a key role in forming and reinforcing popular attitudes about health care, including nursing. So it's not surprising that many people still believe nurses are low-skilled physician assistants rather than college-educated professionals who save lives. In fact, given what people see every day in the media, it would be surprising if most were *not* convinced that health care revolves around brilliant, commanding physicians. This misportrayal undermines the work of all the health professionals who make up the modern health care team, including social workers, physical therapists, and respiratory therapists. In particular, physician-centric media undermines nursing practice and education. And that, in the end, costs lives.

How did the media get so far from the reality of nursing?

# VIRTUE AND VICE:
# SOME ROOTS OF OUR MEDIA STEREOTYPES

Nursing's popular image has long veered among one-dimensional visions of femininity: the angel, the handmaiden, the harlot, or the battle-axe. All these stereotypes can be traced back to the roots of modern nursing, in which groups of nineteenth-century females began trying to help patients with their most intimate problems at times of great stress. But it's worth taking a brief look at the development of nursing image's since then. In doing so, we rely in part on scholars Beatrice and Philip Kalisch, who produced an insightful body of research in the 1980s on the history of the nursing image.[3]

Men and women have long cared for the sick in religious and other settings, as we explained in chapter 1. But in the period just before the founding of modern nursing, the work was regarded as unskilled drudgery unfit for a respectable person. Nursing was consigned to the likes of the immoral, alcohol-abusing Sairey Gamp in Dickens's *Martin Chuzzlewit*.

Florence Nightingale and her fellow reformers changed that. Kalisch and Kalisch describe the era from Nightingale's mid-nineteenth-century work in the Crimea until the end of World War I as one defined by a female "angel of mercy" image. In this period, popular media tended to see nursing as a noble calling, associated it with the military, and regarded nurses themselves with reverence. Some American World War I films featured nurses who volunteered for war duty to be near their soldier boyfriends, then ended up nursing their wounded sweethearts back to health. Kalisch and Kalisch observe that this theme provided a way "to mask the novelty of female independence with traditional female values."

From the 1920s until the end of World War II, nurses were generally seen as pragmatic, even heroic, particularly in war films. The film *A Farewell to Arms* (1932) presented nurses as noble but relatively unskilled, with strict supervisors who enforced a moral code and deference to physicians. The Dr. Kildare films of the 1930s and 1940s focused on an idealized young physician. Nurse characters were young love interests or formidable veterans. Kildare also had a crusty, brilliant diagnostician mentor — a forerunner to House, perhaps. Hitchcock's *Rear Window* (1954) included a late example of what Kalisch and Kalisch describe as this era's "private nurse as detective" portrayals. In the film, the older "insurance company nurse" Stella helps the lovely lead characters unravel a mystery. Stella says she is not well educated, but she is autonomous, quick-witted, and tough.

From the end of World War II until the sixties, nurses tended to be portrayed as maternal helpers to essentially omniscient male physicians. The television show *Ben Casey* (1961–66), for instance, focused on an idealistic young physician not unlike Kildare. The show's nurse character Miss Wills was motherly and relatively unskilled. *Marcus Welby* (1969–76) presented physicians as giving all meaningful care, including even the emotional "caring" that many nurses have traditionally regarded as their area. Kalisch and Kalisch refer to depictions of physicians doing everything as "Marcus Welby syndrome," a malady that is now endemic in Hollywood. According to scholar Joseph Turow, in the 1950s and 1960s the American Medical Association (AMA) asserted control over network television shows, actually vetting scripts. The AMA helpfully ensured that heroic physician characters generally made no errors and lived virtuous lives. Nurses were insignificant.

A few products of the era did focus on nurses. A series of juvenile novels appearing from the 1940s to the 1960s featured Cherry Ames, a virtuous, adventurous, and bright young nurse who moved from job to job solving mysteries (*Cherry Ames: Army Nurse* was a typical title). Cherry Ames inspired many young women to become nurses. A TV series called *The Nurses* (1962–65) actually focused on two hospital nurses, a senior mentor and an inexperienced young nurse. The program even hired a nurse adviser to help the producers develop the show. But already some parents were discouraging talented, ambitious girls from entering nursing.

Then came the sixties. Sexual liberation and expanding work opportunities for women did not enhance public regard for nursing. As many ambitious women began to contemplate careers in medicine and other fields, the nursing image fled back to the poles of extreme female stereotypes. Naughty nurses became a staple of pornography and exploitation films by B-movie king Roger Corman and others. At times, the free-love nurse characters were balanced with senior battle-axes.

Of course, the most notorious example was Nurse Ratched of *One Flew Over the Cuckoo's Nest* (1975). Milos Forman's film adaptation of Ken Kesey's anti-authoritarian 1963 novel featured the senior nurse as a sociopath who abuses her professional and institutional power over her patients. The film is deeply misogynist — every female character is a stereotype — with Ratched as a horrific vision of society's repressed Mom.

Robert Altman's antiwar film *M*A*S*H* (1970), based on Richard Hooker's 1968 novel, was less extreme. But it still presented senior U.S. Army nurse "Hot Lips" Houlihan and other nurses as battle-axes, sex objects, and/or handmaidens to cynical but gifted surgeons during the Korean War. The portrayal of nurses on the influential *M*A*S*H* TV show (1972–83) was somewhat more evolved. The show still focused on the male physicians, who were nicer versions of the film characters: irreverent, gifted leaders trying to save lives in impossible situations — a model for countless future shows. Nurses were often casual sex objects who were there to hand the surgeons things, and Houlihan was a repressed martinet, though she did become far more human, and she displayed some skill and autonomy.

In the 1980s and 1990s, most TV shows presented nurses as peripheral assistants to the dominant physicians, some of whom were now female. A few shows managed to suggest something of what nursing really was. The influential *St. Elsewhere* (1982–88) depicted a fairly gritty Boston hospital. The show's physicians were flawed, but they were still the focus, with the occasional formidable nurse character. *China Beach* (1988–91) was set on a U.S. military base in Vietnam during the Vietnam War. Lead character Colleen McMurphy was a competent, fairly tough Army nurse, but she did not generally display much skill, and the show was mainly about non-health subjects. The minor sitcom *Nurses* (1991–94) treated nurses with some respect. But the notorious *Nightingales* (1988–89) featured sexy but vacuous nursing students who spent so much time in states of partial undress that outraged nurses actually managed to chase the show off the air — a historic anomaly.

*ER* (1994–present) is one of the most influential health care shows in history. It has relied on intense, fairly realistic scenes from a tough Chicago ED and the romantic interactions of roughly ten major characters. *ER* has also presented some of the best depictions of nursing ever to appear on network TV, occasionally showing serious nursing skill and even autonomy. But on the whole it has featured an evolved handmaiden image: nurses are skilled physician assistants who must ultimately defer. The show has never had more than one major nurse character at a time, and it has always relied heavily on physician nursing. Like Marcus Welby, *ER* physicians save lives using traditional medical skills *and* provide virtually all important bedside care, including key psychosocial care.

At the turn of the millennium, a few other shows had nurse characters of some substance, though no show challenged the idea that only physicians really matter. The Lifetime drama *Strong Medicine* (2000–2006) included hunky, articulate nurse midwife Peter Riggs, a progressive underling set against the female physician stars — probably a model for Dell from *Private Practice*. But the show's other nurses were mute handmaidens. The kooky sitcom *Scrubs* (2001–present) has featured tough nurse Carla Espinosa, who has at times displayed real skill. But the show's physicians provide virtually all important care, and the nurses are generally assistants without compelling or accurate story lines.

Today the state of the art for Hollywood nursing portrayals is clearly the peripheral, low-skilled physician handmaiden with virtually nothing to contribute. *Grey's Anatomy* and *House* remain massively popular. Every major character on these shows is a physician, and the shows' vision of nursing is that of a job in a sad time warp. Now that female physicians are so common, there's no need to include nurse characters at all to have a gender mix that is good for drama. The subtext is obvious: today, no person of substance would even *think* of becoming a nurse. Those who do are pathetic losers unworthy of a second glance from TV viewers. Or even a first glance: let's just show their forearms at the edge of the frame, holding something for the pretty, smart physicians.

# DOES WHAT'S IN OUR BRAINS MATTER? HOW THE MEDIA INFLUENCES NURSING

At this point, you may be wondering how media portrayals of nurses affect the profession. The Center for Nursing Advocacy often receives skeptical letters on this subject. Here are some of the questions we receive, and our replies.

*Come on. Even if the media ignores nursing or presents it inaccurately, how can that possibly affect nursing in real life?*

What people see and hear affects what they think. And what they think affects what they do. This is a basic principle of education, religion, art, and any other organized effort to influence people. It is why major corporations spend millions on advertising campaigns to promote their products, and why powerful political ads can move polling numbers and affect election results.

The same principle applies to health issues. Indeed, in recent years a consensus has emerged in the field of public health that the media affects society's health-related views and behavior. Public agencies, private groups, and scholars now devote substantial resources to analyzing and managing health messages in the media.

The field of health communications addresses how this works. As public health scholar Deborah Glik noted in "Health Communication in Popular Media Formats" (2003), media products "comprise both planned and unplanned content which has the potential to communicate positive, neutral or negative health messages to the public."[4] The inclusion of "unplanned" content means the media influences people whether or not the creators *intended* it, just as a parent may influence a child in a certain way without intending to. The media need not intend to harm nursing to have that effect.

Glik has noted that "from a social marketing perspective, messages in the media that promote specific desirable behaviors have the potential to persuade consumers to change their behavior if messages are viewed as compatible with consumers' own self-interest, competing messages are minimal, and resistance to change is low to moderate." And it makes little sense to think that people would learn about substantive health topics like cancer or AIDS from a media product but form no opinions about the health worker who is presenting the information.

In a 2002 report to the Kaiser Family Foundation, scholars Joseph Turow and Rachel Gans noted that "researchers have long recognized that news media coverage affects what the public believes about health care."[5] Advocates have therefore worked hard to affect the media's coverage of health topics in which they have an interest.

For example, as Turow, Suzanne Gordon, and Bernice Buresh have shown, physicians have worked hard for decades to manage their public image. We have noted that the AMA has historically tried to control how physicians are depicted in the media. It has also aggressively promoted coverage of medical research and other physician-centered stories. In general, these efforts have been a resounding success. Research has confirmed that physicians, a critical part of the health care team, are generally portrayed by the news media as more or less the *whole* team. Physicians are often consulted on issues, such as nutrition and breastfeeding, in which others generally have as much if not greater expertise. Physicians' combination of economic, social, and moral status is unrivaled by any other professional group.

Public health scholars try to increase understanding of what the media is saying, sometimes subtly, about health issues. Glik has explained that, "given the pervasiveness and potential power of the media to shape beliefs, attitudes and behaviors, the media literacy movement has emerged." This movement aims to help children and teens understand what the media is really doing, but these skills are also important for adults, especially those whose interests are not served by current media practice. Glik describes the popular media as a "double-edged sword" that may function "as both a tool for progress and a source of ill health that is a reflection of the larger culture it represents."

In particular, we must explore how the media affects one of the most important global health problems: the crisis in nursing. When those without much understanding of nursing get a lifetime of negative stereotypical messages about the profession, they do not consider nursing as a career. Likewise, public officials and health care decision makers with little understanding of nursing's real importance do not allocate sufficient funds for nurse staffing, nursing education, or nursing research. And nurses themselves are not immune. The media's undervaluation can sap nurses' pride, encourage cynicism and self-loathing, and discourage nurses from standing up for themselves and their patients.

On the whole, the nursing crisis can be seen as the result of an entire society's failing to value nursing adequately. But the media is a key factor in that failure.

*OK, I can see that some media probably affect how people think about and act toward nursing, like maybe a newspaper article. But how can some TV drama, sitcom, or commercial affect people that way? People don't take that stuff seriously!*

The effects of fictional media are not always obvious, but they have been felt throughout history in every culture, from Homer to Homer Simpson. These effects have been recognized as important by the health community, the news media, and even Hollywood. And today, more fictional media are more available to more of the world's people than ever before.

To believe that we can disregard everything we perceive in the entertainment media because the scenarios presented aren't literally "true," we would also have to believe that people disregard all messages in advertising, since ads often present actors in simulated situations. But that is not how our minds work.

In a recent TV ad for the Dodge Caravan minivan, a female OR "nurse" asks a female "brain surgeon" which of two scalpels she wants. The surgeon confidently explains which one she needs. Then, in response to a similarly phrased question from the nurse, the surgeon practically commands the nurse to buy a Caravan rather than an SUV. The ad also features a goofy male anesthesia professional and a dopey male patient (who drives an SUV). Later, the surgeon picks up her kids with the Caravan. The voiceover notes that it "doesn't take a brain surgeon" to know that there's "no smarter choice."

We know we are not seeing real OR workers. But that does not stop us from absorbing the messages embedded in this clever ad. Despite being fiction, the ad might influence our views of the vehicle, of the ability of women to become authoritative professionals, and of the knowledge and roles of physicians and nurses. Some of this result may be "unplanned," but all of it sells the minivan to the target demographic, which is presumably working mothers. Most people would probably admit that this ad has some positive influence on society's overall view of women. But that is because there is broad social understanding that women can now become esteemed professionals. Nursing is not well understood, and society has little basis to question the subtext that the brain surgeon is "smarter" than the submissive nurse about health care (and everything else).

The idea that fictional media can influence public views and conduct is not controversial in the field of public health. In their 2002 Kaiser Report, Turow and Gans conclude that "fictional television can [] play a significant role in shaping public images about the state of our health care system and policy options for improving the delivery of care." Glik agrees that "an important aspect of health communications today is working with the entertainment media to include or improve health messages in popular programs." A 2004 Kaiser Family Foundation Report confirmed that "many groups have come to believe that entertainment media can play an important positive role in educating the public about significant health messages."[6] Conversely, Glik notes that a good deal of ongoing research has found "unhealthy messages" in entertainment media, for instance smoking in films, which Glik reports has been shown to influence rates of teen smoking.

Turow and Gans explain why entertainment television may actually influence views of health care *even more* than the news media does:

> Certainly TV dramas reach a much wider audience than most news programs. Beyond the size of their audience, some media scholars argue that entertainment TV's impact can be even more powerful than news in subtly shaping the public's impressions of key societal institutions. The messages are more engaging, often playing out in compelling human dramas involving characters the audience cares about. Viewers are taken behind the scenes to see the hidden forces affecting whether there's a happy ending or a sad one. There are good guys and bad guys, heroes and villains and innocent bystanders. Instead of bill numbers and budget figures, policy issues

are portrayed through the lives of "real" human beings, often in life-and-death situations. These health policy discussions take place not only in hospital dramas, but also in dramatic storylines on programs like "Law and Order," "The Practice," and "The West Wing."

Hospital dramas provide an opportunity for viewers to learn specifically what goes on at the center of high-intensity medicine. The dramas' fictional presentations open curtains on relationships between doctors and nurses, specialists and generalists. In ways that news reports cannot, they play out various assumptions about how health care ought to be delivered, about what conflicts arise that affect health care, and about how those conflicts should be resolved and why. Doing that, hospital dramas represent an important part of viewers' curriculum on the problems and possibilities of health care in America.

Even more to the point, Turow and Gans stress that TV hospital dramas' "consistent focus on the relation of doctors and nurses with patients who are in jeopardy make them the source of many viewers' understandings of how the health care system works."

Because of the great influence of entertainment media, Turow and Gans note, public health organizations everywhere "are increasingly turning to entertainment media — from soap operas to sitcoms to reality shows — as a way to reach the public with health messages." This growing effort is often called "entertainment education." Glik defines it as "a way of informing the public about a social issue or concern" by "incorporating an educational message into popular entertainment content in order to raise awareness, increase knowledge, create favorable attitudes, and ultimately motivate people to take socially responsible action in their own lives." Much entertainment education results from what the 2004 Kaiser Report describes as "outreach efforts of special interest groups or health agencies to deliver their message to audiences. These groups often work with Hollywood-based advocacy organizations that serve as liaisons to the entertainment community via industry forums, roundtable briefings, and technical script consultations."

Among the organizations devoting significant resources to entertainment education in recent years are the Harvard and UCLA schools of public health. In addition, the Hollywood, Health & Society project at the University of Southern California has collaborated with producers of prime-time shows and soap operas to place messages on a wide variety of health topics, including infectious diseases, diabetes, and health care access. This project is a joint venture whose sponsors include the Centers for Disease Control and Prevention (CDC), and the Writers Guild of America. And the Kaiser Family Foundation has worked with various Hollywood shows to place health messages and story lines on subjects including emergency contraception and teen sexual activity.

The health community's entertainment education efforts are not confined to the developed world. A December 2004 Associated Press story described a Cambodian soap opera created by British soap guru Matthew Robinson and funded by the BBC World Service Trust to educate Cambodians about disease, especially HIV/AIDS. *Taste of Life* reportedly "follows five student nurses and a student doctor as they move through a nursing college, the local pub and 'Friendship Hospital.'"

On the other hand, public health scholars confirm that Hollywood shows can also cause real harm. Purdue communications professor Susan Morgan is the co-author of recent research suggesting that negative entertainment TV portrayals of organ donation (including on *Grey's Anatomy*) have contributed to negative views about the vital health practice. Morgan is quoted in a September 2007 *Forbes* article: "It's hard not to get kind of outraged when you see what's going on. You could start drawing this out to real human lives being lost."

Though Hollywood is reluctant to admit that its products can cause harm, the industry embraces the idea that it can have a *positive* effect on public health. Indeed, many Hollywood figures seem proud to have improved health through entertainment. In presenting former *ER* producer (and physician) Neal Baer with a public service award in December 2003, the Writers Guild of America lauded him for "creating a culture of medical accuracy and groundbreaking realism that revolutionized the primetime landscape." The WGA also asserted that the producer's "passion for medical accuracy has paid dividends to the American public, as a recent Harvard study revealed most Americans learn more about health-related problems from series television like *Law and Order: Special Victims Unit* than from their own doctors." Baer, in addition to executive-producing *SVU*, is co-chair of the advisory board of Hollywood, Health & Society. Likewise, in a 2004 issue of *TV Guide*, a medical adviser and an executive producer from *ER* were eager to celebrate the show's apparent influence on the number of women pursuing emergency medicine. And in a 2005 NPR interview, *Grey's* creator Shonda Rhimes stressed that her show could help people of color, because "the way people look at people on television is the way they perceive the world. And for me the idea of the show, part of it, is that we can change the assumptions that people have simply by the images they see in the background of the show."

Sadly, those who proclaim the *positive* health effects of Hollywood shows seem unwilling to consider how the industry's inaccurate depiction of nurses as peripheral subordinates could have *negative* effects. Though there is no dispute that the shows affect social views and knowledge of disease, viewers must have some innate filter that blocks even the most compelling media information about health workers' professional roles.

In fact, as we have shown, physicians have long understood the power of entertainment media. In their article "Doc Hollywood" (2001), Gordon and Buresh cite the "symbiotic relationship" physicians have with Hollywood, which "has been an active partner in the creation of a heroic medical narrative that has shaped Americans' view of health care…and conferred status on medical practitioners and specialists."[6] Today, physicians provide virtually all significant expert health care advice for entertainment programming. Nurses may be on set adjusting minor technical details, but physicians are the ones who consult regularly on the scripts that actually drive the shows. Indeed, *ER* was created by physician Michael Crichton, and a number of its key writers have been physicians. At least one *House* writer is a physician. The creator of *Scrubs* based the show on the experiences of one of his best friends, a physician who advises the show.

Recently news articles have addressed how entertainment programming affects viewers' health-related actions. In October 2006, the *Orange County Register* ran Lisa Liddane's "Paging Dr. Nielsen: TV medical shows." The piece examined how popular hospital dramas like *Grey's Anatomy* reflect and shape real-life health matters. Producers, physician writers, and public health experts confirmed that although such shows are fiction, they affect what the public thinks about health care. Vicky Rideout of the Kaiser Family Foundation noted that "TV medical dramas contribute to agenda-setting — and influence how people look at situations and professions."[7]

In late 2006 and early 2007, a slew of similar and increasingly high-profile articles followed the *Register* piece. In every case, the discussion among writers, physicians, and public health advocates focused on the extent to which the shows' technical portrayal of medical conditions was accurate. None mentioned the generally abysmal portrayal of nursing. A March 2007 article in *Reader's Digest*, Mary A. Fischer's "Docs in the Box," spent a great deal of time on "medical authenticity." The piece mentioned one nurse: *Grey's* consultant Linda Klein. Star Ellen Pompeo assured readers Klein "takes the time to show us exactly how something should be done." That is, the nurse consultant shows the actors playing physicians how to do important things nurses really do, and lends an air of realism to a show that portrays her profession as trivial scut work.

In the first half of 2007, a few articles at last focused on the inaccuracy of the nursing portrayals on these shows. Carol Ann Campbell's excellent "Nurses Urge TV Dramas: Get Real," in the New Jersey *Star-Ledger* in January 2007, had nurses explain how TV dramas regularly show physicians doing important work that nurses really do, while showing nurses as peripheral subordinates. The piece suggested that this misrepresentation contributes to the shortage of nurses. Similar articles followed in several smaller papers. The *Star-Ledger* managed to get *House* creator David Shore to comment. Shore admitted his show "ignores" nurses but noted that the character House treats everyone badly. In fact, the show treats nurses in the same contemptuous way House does, and has made virtually no effort to rebut any of House's slurs. Shore even resorted to noting that his mother is a nurse and she "loves" the show.[8]

In September 2007 *Forbes* ran Allison Van Dusen's "Playing Doctor: Medical TV Isn't Always Right." The piece addressed the overall accuracy and effects of popular health-related TV dramas — *and* discussed the concerns of nurses. It even pointed out that nurse characters tend to absorb abuse from physicians like House with no ability to respond, reinforcing the image of nurses as meek servants.[9]

This is an era of media saturation, diverse content, and technological development — an age of virtual reality. It is increasingly difficult to tell what is "real." There is little doubt that today's "fictional" media profoundly affects how we think and act.

*Fine, I get that public health scholars, physicians, and even Hollywood believes the entertainment media affects real world health. But does any recent research say so?*

Recent research has shown that entertainment television has a clear and powerful effect on viewers' health-related thoughts — and actions. This influence flows not only from prime-time dramas like *Grey's Anatomy* and *ER* but even from sitcoms and soap operas.

Some limited research has addressed Hollywood's poor nursing portrayal. Most notably, in 2000 the ad agency JWT Communications conducted a focus group study of 1,800 youngsters in grades two through ten; respondents said they received their main impression of nursing from *ER*. They knew more about the nurses' love lives than their professional work. Consistent with the show's physician-centric approach, the young people wrongly said nursing was a girl's job, that it was a technical job "like shop," and that it was not a career for private school students, of whom more was expected.[10] And in their 2002 Kaiser Report, Turow and Gans reported that their research had found that physicians dominated discussions of health policy issues on U.S. hospital dramas, while nurses hardly appeared.

More generally, when the U.S. Centers for Disease Control and Prevention surveyed prime-time TV viewers in 2000, they found that most (52 percent) reported getting information that they trust to be accurate from prime-time TV shows. More than a quarter said such shows were among their top three sources for health information. Nine out of ten regular viewers said they learned something about diseases from television, with almost half citing prime-time or daytime entertainment shows. Moreover, almost half of regular viewers who heard something about a health issue on a prime-time show said they took one or more actions, including telling someone about the story line (42 percent), telling someone to do something or doing it themselves, such as using a condom or getting more exercise (16 percent), or visiting a clinic or physician (9 percent).[11]

Recent research has also shown that entertainment shows influence public views of specific areas of health care. One 2007 study published in *Health Communication* found that organ donation was presented in a negative or inaccurate way in the great majority of plotlines in fictional prime-time and daytime shows (including comedies and soap operas) in 2004 and 2005.[12] A 2005 study published in *Clinical Transplantation* likewise found that most organ donation plotlines were flawed, and that respondents who had negative views of organ donation often mentioned what they'd seen on TV as a basis for their opinions. And a 2007 study by Yale researchers published in the journal *Plastic and Reconstructive Surgery* found that plastic surgery reality shows played an important role in patients' knowledge and decisions about the procedures.[13]

Some research has focused on the effects of specific shows. In September 2008, the Kaiser Family Foundation released a study showing that an embedded *Grey's Anatomy* plotline about maternal HIV transmission had significantly increased audience understanding of the issue.[14] The show's own "director of medical research" helped to publicize the study, and she told *TV Guide* that the show took its influence "very seriously."

Many studies have documented the long-running *ER*'s effects on views about health care. In addition to the JWT focus group study, a 1998 article in the *Journal of the American Medical Association* concluded that medical students' reactions to shows like *ER* suggested that the students "may incorporate the attitudes and beliefs of physicians on television in much the same way they acquire the qualities and behaviors of physicians through their experiences in patient care." The article cited other research showing the dramatic growth in ED medical residencies since *ER*'s premiere a few years earlier.[15] A Kaiser Family Foundation survey found that more than half of those who were regular *ER* viewers during the 1997–2000 seasons said they learned about important health issues while watching the show. Almost a third said information from the show helped them make choices about their family's health care. Almost a quarter had sought further information about a health issue, and 14 percent had actually contacted a health care provider because of something they saw in an *ER* episode. And according to a 2001 Kaiser Foundation National Survey of Physicians, "one in five doctors say they are consulted 'very' or 'somewhat' often about specific diseases or treatments that patients heard about on TV shows such as 'ER.'"[16]

*ER* also affects what viewers think about specific conditions. In September 2007, University of Southern California researchers published a study in the *Journal of Health Communication* that found those who saw an *ER* plotline about teen obesity and hypertension were 65 percent more likely to report that they had acted in a healthier way.[17] A 2002 study at the Harvard School of Public Health found that regular *ER* viewers were far more aware (57 versus 39 percent) of the need to get a smallpox vaccination right after exposure following an episode dealing with the subject.[18]

Entertainment media does not have to be mainly about health care to affect viewers' understanding of health care issues. In 2002 a RAND Health survey of regular viewers of the sitcom *Friends* aged twelve to seventeen found that respondents retained important information from a story line depicting an unplanned pregnancy caused by condom failure. The report concluded that "entertainment television can be most effective as an educator when teens and parents view together and discuss what they watch."[19]

The effects of health-related entertainment programming are also not confined to popular prime-time shows. In 1999 a CDC survey "found that many daytime viewers also report learning about health issues from TV." Almost half of regular daytime drama viewers reported learning something about a disease from watching soap operas. Over one-third reported taking some action after hearing about a health issue or disease on a soap opera.[20] And a 2004 study published in the *Journal of Communication* found that after an episode of *The Bold and the Beautiful* with an HIV subplot, and subsequent display of the CDC's National STD and AIDS hotline, calls to the hotline spiked.[21]

A May/June 2008 *Nursing Economics* study confirmed that the media affects public understanding of nursing—although the article claimed that nursing is "highly respected."[22] The 2007 public opinion research on which the article relied was funded by drug company Johnson & Johnson (J&J), which had been faulted for airing television recruiting ads promoting an unskilled angel image of nursing. One question asked respondents whether certain broad categories of media made them "respect" nurses more or less. A category consisting of the television shows *ER*, *Scrubs*, *House*, and *Grey's Anatomy* reportedly made no difference to 66 percent of respondents but made 28 percent respect nurses more, and only 5 percent respect nurses less.

The vague category "advertisements about nursing" — which presumably included the J&J ads — had no effect on 60 percent, but supposedly created more respect in 38 percent and less in only 1 percent. In fact, *none* of the media tested had a large negative effect. Evidently, either *every* class of media creates positive views of nurses, or else only the positive media affects people. The *Nursing Economics* survey was too vague and subject to self-reporting bias to provide much useful data. Respondents are unlikely to admit to a pollster that the media makes them "respect" real nurses less. Most people know they're supposed to honor nurses in the abstract. But this generalized affection has not translated into the resources that would show real respect for nurses as professionals. "Respect" can mean different things: is it respect for nurses' life-saving skills, or for their hearts of gold? And the study failed to reconcile its results with what the media it tested actually said about nursing.

In any case, this wealth of research shows that entertainment programming is easily "realistic" enough to affect real world health care — including nursing.

*Well, if all that research shows how influential Hollywood is, why won't the industry improve its damaging portrayal of nursing?*

So far Hollywood's responses have been inadequate. The industry argues that Hollywood shows are not documentaries and producers must have "dramatic license"; that entertainment media has to focus on physicians because that's what viewers want; that it's just a mean central character who hates nurses, the show really loves them; that there was a shortage of nurses before their show came on the air; that nurses *do* advise the show and they work on set ensuring "medical accuracy"; and that the show works hard to present an accurate portrayal of all health professionals. But none of that has prevented the industry from offering hundreds of hours of damaging misportrayals of nursing.

The factors underlying Hollywood's overall failure to portray nursing fairly are complex and varied. In our view, they include:

- entrenched stereotypes about nursing that persist even among the educated media elite, despite the increasing scope and complexity of modern nursing care;

- Hollywood's reliance on conventions and its fairly light focus on the complex realities of society compared to the focus of the news media, which is trained to at least try to report what it actually sees, rather than just what its audience expects to see;

- the fact that nursing remains overwhelmingly female, while men still control most Hollywood programming, and that nursing has not generally enjoyed the respect or understanding of media "feminists" with the power to effect change;

- insufficient support from physicians, who are often the beneficiaries of the misportrayal of nursing, and who provide virtually all meaningful health care advice in Hollywood;

- nursing's own overall failure to represent itself well to the media and the public at large, as explained in Buresh and Gordon's *From Silence to Voice*;

- the failure of nurses' concerns, even when assertively presented, to be taken as seriously as the concerns of other groups, perhaps owing to the Catch-22 of the poor image itself: why pay attention to nurses when they're just unskilled handmaidens?; and

- "PC fatigue" and an apparent belief among "progressive" media creators that their work has a positive social impact (such as on race and gender issues), immunizing them from responsibility for other ills.

At one time, health care media creators might have felt they had to include nurses to get a good gender mix and good drama. But today, with so many female physicians, most media creators evidently feel that they need not include any significant nurse characters at all. And on network television, once all your main characters are physicians, the need to constantly sell those characters means they're going to be doing everything, regardless of what happens in real life.

You might think physicians, who wield so much power in Hollywood, would have a better sense of nursing. Some physicians do. But much physician conduct seems to reflect a narrow, internally focused approach that assumes physicians provide all important health care and need not consider unexpected information. Physicians in general know little about nursing. Some physicians have even said that nurses get "too much education" and that they could "train monkeys" to do nurses' jobs.

*But don't nurses bear some responsibility for the poor understanding of their profession?*

Yes, of course. But we focus on the media's treatment of nursing because it is wildly inaccurate and distorted. Millions are given access to the lives and work of nurses through the media, so the media plays an enormous role in shaping and reinforcing social beliefs, as public health research shows. The popular media also provides an excellent vehicle to engage the public's interest. The media presents a set of common social reference points in which large parts of the world public already have a deep interest.

Nursing itself has many problems. Far from trying to substitute a positive stereotype of nurses for the negative ones, we simply want people to look at nurses as they really are. We also recognize that nurses often do not present themselves in an ideal way; we discuss this in chapter 11. From major nursing institutions that continue to embrace unskilled "angel" imagery ("Nurses have a passion for caring!"), to nurses who welcome the idea that people will assess them professionally by how "hot" they are, to nurses who won't speak up in clinical or public settings about the work they really do, to nurses who show the Hollywood actors playing physicians how to do things nurses really do — there is plenty of responsibility to go around.

Solving nursing's problems will require a range of strategies. Improving public understanding is one of the most important.

*But that television show just happens to be about physicians. Even if it might help nursing to include nurses, how can you expect the show to do that?*

In 2008, twenty-eight of twenty-nine major characters on the top three U.S. hospital dramas just "happened" to be physicians. And in all these hospital shows, in hundreds of hours of programming seen by millions around the world, the physician characters just "happened" to spend half their time doing key tasks that nurses do in real life. These are not random phenomena. We see no sign that things will soon even out, that such shows will spend many years with 95 percent nurse characters, who will spend lots of time on tasks physicians really do. Today's health care media landscape reflects a critical lack of understanding and widespread social bias.

What seems to just "happen" in Hollywood is actually driven by the vast gulf between what media creators think and how things really are. In Hollywood, physicians single-handedly save lives. In real life, nurses also save countless lives. In Hollywood, physicians do virtually all critical procedures, like defibrillation. In real life, nurses perform many critical procedures, including most defibrillations. In Hollywood, physicians stay with patients 24/7, providing monitoring, emotional support, and education. In real life, nurses do that. In Hollywood, nurses are mute, deferential physician servants. In real life, they are autonomous professionals with years of college-level education who play the central role in hospitals. Their work is challenging and exciting, and they use their advanced skills to improve patient outcomes every day, often with little or no involvement from physicians.

*Sorry, but even if media stereotypes do undermine nursing, I just don't see why I should care. What's in it for me?*

You get to live. People sometimes ask journalist Suzanne Gordon why she, not a nurse, has worked so hard to publicize the roots of the nursing crisis and potential solutions. Her response is that it's enlightened self-interest: she wants someone to be there to care for her when she needs it. Too few nurses leads to worse patient outcomes, suffering, and death.

The effects of the undervaluation of nursing are everywhere. When nurses lack resources, patients do not receive vital care. When nurses lack resources, they burn out and leave the bedside. When nurses lack social power, they cannot advocate for patients, and patients die needlessly from medical errors and incompetence. A December 2007 Associated Press article reported that OR nurses at a Rhode Island hospital had repeatedly failed to stop life-threatening surgical errors — like operating on the wrong side of a patient's head — because they lacked the social power to do so.

When nurses lack social power, they also suffer abuse from colleagues and patients. U.S. nurses are assaulted more often than prison guards, and little is done about it. A 2008 study by the Joint Commission on the Accreditation of Healthcare Organizations found that more than half of U.S. nurses had been bullied on the job.[23] Common effects included severe distress, depression, insomnia — and nurses themselves continuing the cycle of abuse.

These are the people who hold your life in their hands.

# PART TWO

# The Great Divide:
# The Media versus Real Nursing

# CHAPTER 3

# Could Monkeys Be Nurses?

NBC's CAMPY DAYTIME drama *Passions* offered a very special solution to the nursing shortage: an orangutan. From 2003 until 2005, viewers could watch the monkey play the role of Precious, a private duty nurse. Character Beth Wallace hired Precious to replace her invalid mother's previous nurse, who had blabbed Beth's secrets.

The NBC website told us the "dutiful caretaker" changed Mrs. Wallace's diapers, wore "a modern version of a nurse's uniform, complete with cap," adored "handsome Latino men, bananas, fruit smoothies, shopping, food fights, gin and tonics," and wanted "to do the best job possible as Mrs. Wallace's nurse...and to have some fun at the same time!"

While *Passions* was known for being completely over the top, the role of Precious reflects public sentiment about the work of nurses. There are those who believe nursing requires so little skill that a monkey *could* do it. In fact, in the 1990s, representatives of a California hospital group told top-level union negotiators that nursing was so simple the union's nurses could be replaced with monkeys.

This chapter explores how recent media has portrayed nursing skill. A number of media items, particularly in print news, have communicated some sense of the advanced scientific skills that nurses use to improve patient outcomes. Unfortunately, much of the most influential media, particularly television, regularly sends the message that nursing is low-skilled loser work unworthy of serious consideration by anyone with a brain.

In addition, countless media items portray important nursing work as being performed by others, particularly physicians, thus robbing nurses of credit they need to save their profession. Others ignore nursing work and expertise, even when nursing actually plays a central role in the relevant subject, such as patient education, managing health care errors, or mass casualty events. Still other items suggest that any helpful person or machine is a "nurse," consistent with the broad use of the term "nursing" to include unskilled tending.

The prevailing view of nursing as inferior grunt work undermines nurses' claims to respect and resources. In a May 2008 *Arab News* article, Taqwa Omer Yahia, a nursing dean at Saudi Arabia's King Saud University, described what happened when she gave a lecture at a local university. She was introduced as "Dr. Yahia" and "treated with respect and admiration" until, after her talk, a student asked "what kind of doctor" she was. Dr. Yahia said that her PhD was in nursing. The students' disappointment was palpable, and she felt she had "lost all credibility as a trusted speaker."

The orangutan Nurse Precious reminds us of a study Harvard researchers once did. In the study, participants watched a small circle of people throw basketballs to each other. As the basketballs went back and forth, a person dressed in a gorilla costume walked into the middle of the circle, stopped to beat her chest, and left the circle. But most observers later reported seeing nothing unusual. They did not see the "gorilla" because they were not expecting to see it.[1] In the same way, most of us have trouble seeing what nurses *really* do because we are conditioned to see only what we *think* they do.

## MEDIA PORTRAYALS OF NURSES AS SERIOUS PROFESSIONALS

Portrayals of nurses as skilled professionals do exist. They tend to appear in the print news media, but it is possible to find them even on entertainment television. Nurses have been portrayed as skilled clinicians, vital public health workers, researchers and innovators, health care experts and leaders, and just as important, as people whose work is serious enough that death can result when it isn't done right.

### "Excuse Me, Miss Peyton": Nursing Skill on Television and in Film

Relatively realistic portrayals of nursing skill have sometimes appeared on *ER*. Typically, these involve the lone major nurse character, who in recent years has been the tough, competent Samantha (Sam) Taggart. Of course, the show has also denigrated nursing skill, offered rampant physician nursing, and shown nurses reporting to physicians. But it is far better than other dramas, inserting at least passing indications of nursing skill and knowledge.

A handful of late 2005 *ER* episodes featured hard-core nurse manager Eve Peyton. Peyton was the only significant nurse character the show portrayed as a clinical peer of the attending physicians. October 2005 episodes showed her taking the ED nursing staff firmly in hand, mentoring nurse Taggart, and pushing back against senior physicians. In one scene, busy attending Luka Kovac repeatedly brushed off Peyton's requests that he come to an adjoining trauma room to help a flailing resident with a fiberoptic intubation for a hypoxic accident victim with severe head trauma. Peyton picked up the difficult airway box and headed out of the room. Kovac, sensing trouble, began, "Excuse me, Miss Peyton — " Peyton told him that she had a PhD, so if he wanted to get formal, he could call her "Doctor."

When Kovac managed to get next door, the resident and the rest of the code team were watching Peyton insert a laryngeal mask airway, educating as she went. The patient quickly improved. Peyton suggested that Kovac consider educating his residents about using the LMA to rescue can't-intubate/can't-ventilate patients. The patient's mother tearfully thanked Peyton, who told Kovac, "Take it from here, Doctor. I'm going to go find a bedpan that needs emptying." Although the physician characters still dominated care in the Peyton episodes, Peyton was perhaps the most clinically expert nurse character ever to appear on a major prime-time U.S. show.

A number of other recent *ER* episodes also stand out for depictions of nursing skill. For example, in one February 2007 episode, the physicians had trouble intubating a critical patient. Taggart pushed the sides of the patient's chest to force air back up through the trachea, explaining that "the bubbles will show you where to place the tube." Attending Archie Morris was blown away: "Sam is the man."

The irreverent NBC sitcom *Scrubs* (which moved to ABC in 2008) is similarly dominated by physician characters, but it too has included some passing indications of nursing skill. Most have involved the show's one major nurse character, Carla Espinosa, who at times is presented as a nurse manager. An April 2006 episode showed Espinosa catching intern errors and teaching the interns how to avoid them. In one scene, Espinosa even expertly took charge of handling a patient's seizure, with an intern following her lead. And a minor plotline in a March 2006 episode featured an aggressive defense of nurses' technical expertise, as Espinosa demonstrated her encyclopedic knowledge of the conditions and care plans of specific patients.

A couple Discovery Health Channel documentaries have also given a good sense of nursing skill, though their audience has been limited. *Lifeline: The Nursing Diaries*, a three-part documentary broadcast in 2004, followed the work of nurses at Massachusetts General and New York–Presbyterian hospitals. The first part, "The Rookies," produced by master documentary maker Richard Kahn and Linda Martin, is possibly the best single hour of a nursing documentary that we've seen. It shows highly skilled nursing actions that the media often ignores or assigns to physicians, including life-saving interventions, patient education, and family support in intensive care units. Helen Holt's *Nurses*, broadcast in 2002, was an accurate and engaging five-part documentary following the work of nurses at Johns Hopkins. Episodes focused on oncology, the neonatal intensive care unit, critical care, pediatrics, and psychiatric care.

A few recent feature-length films have conveyed something of nursing skill. Mike Nichols's *Angels in America*, based on Tony Kushner's play, includes one of the best depictions of nursing in feature film history, placing the profession at the center of AIDS care. Shown on HBO in 2003, the six-hour exploration of faith, politics, and sexuality is set at the start of the AIDS era. Belize is a nurse who employs skill, cynical wit, and tough love to keep his stricken friend Prior alive and sane. Meanwhile, Roy Cohn, the corrupt lawyer and conservative power broker, ends up on Belize's AIDS ward.

Belize provides Cohn with a measure of comfort, dignity, and sound advice, even as they trade invective across a chasm of mutual loathing. When Cohn's upper-crust physician Henry comes to have the dying sociopath admitted, he and Belize exchange barbs that reveal something of nurse-physician relations. Henry tells Belize that the new admit is a "very important man." Belize: "Oh, OK, then I shouldn't f--- up his medication?" In addition to Belize, the skilled nurse practitioner Emily appears to direct Prior's outpatient care, monitoring his treatment and helping him confront his fears.

Then there's the 2004 overhaul of George Romero's zombie classic *Dawn of the Dead* by the director Zack Snyder and screenwriter James Gunn. The movie is a funny post-9/11 vision of radical fundamentalism overrunning bourgeois society. Character Ana Clark, a smart, tough, resourceful nurse, helps lead some survivors trapped in a suburban mall. She cares for the group's wounds, uses her nursing skill to discover vital zombie information, and responds to one character's snotty "What are you, a f---ing doctor?" by snapping, "No, I'm a f---ing nurse."

## "Startling Discoveries": Nursing Skill in the News Media

Most effective recent portrayals of nursing skill have appeared in the print press. These do not generally have the broad impact of television or movies, though they may reach influential demographics.

### EXPERTS, LIFE SAVERS, AND LEADERS

In April 2007 the *Wall Street Journal* published a piece by editor John Blanton, who had resigned from the paper, gone back to school, and become a nurse in a post-9/11 search for meaning. Focused on the crushing workload and fear of error Blanton faced as a new burn unit nurse, the article delivered unusually specific descriptions of nursing care. Blanton explained that in his first months, any deviation from "the template of nursing duties [he] had been taught to perform like clockwork" could throw him off.

With easily shattered confidence, I could start an IV, administer medications, bathe a bed-bound patient and change linens, change dressings, insert all sorts of catheters and tubes, read lab results and electrocardiograms. I knew to be vigilant against infection, pneumonia, pressure ulcers, medication errors and the many other lurking threats to hospital patients. On the burn unit, pain control loomed large. I also knew, as both executor of treatment plans and patient advocate, to keep a close eye on what doctors ordered. They make mistakes, too.

Blanton tells us exactly what he did for patients and why it mattered. He hits the daunting stress and workload of his early months hard, but when he gets to some of the satisfaction of being a good nurse — such as a boy's request to be in Blanton's care again — it means far more because we know that he is not an unskilled hand-holder.

In October 2005 the *Boston Globe* ran Scott Allen's four-part special report about the intense eight-month ICU training of new nurse Julia Zelixon by veteran nurse M. J. Pender. Readers got a vivid sense of the complexity and importance of highly skilled nursing. Pender's analysis of the patients' conditions and needs was relentless, as the nurses worked to manage different medications, tubes, and monitors. The ICU training was so hard that four of the seventeen nurses in Zelixon's program would not make it, "a higher dropout rate than basic training for the Marines." Each patient reportedly needed twenty hours of nursing care daily. The piece noted that nurses provide the vast majority of such care on their own. An anesthesiologist pointed to the much higher patient loads of physicians and noted that he often feels "we're here more as consultants to the nurses." At another point, Pender told a resident that a patient would need a nasogastric tube and sent the resident to get it. Pender stopped a physician from speeding a transfusion to an especially critical patient, fearing that it would dilute the medication dripping through the same IV. At one point, it became clear that a young accident victim with an array of serious ailments would soon die. Pender decided that the patient's husband should come in. The piece conveyed her expertise at this delicate task, as she introduced herself, encouraged the husband to take his wife's hand, and cleared the room of nonessential staff.

A July 2007 piece by Chris Colin on the *San Francisco Chronicle* website profiled nurses at the University of California at San Francisco's Neonatal Intensive Care Unit (NICU). The piece discussed nurses' personal qualities, but it also noted that their expertise saves lives.

> Studying their every move means observing startling competence. A Stephen Hawking-ish level of knowledge bounces casually around the unit. (More than once I was convinced they were sprinkling their conversation with purely invented terms. Hemolysis? Cannulation?)

In 2004, Garry Trudeau's widely distributed comic strip *Doonesbury* introduced tough Walter Reed character Nurse Jewel, who cared for Lt. B.D. after he lost part of his leg in the Iraq war. In a June strip, Jewel told B.D. that the hospital's nurses "love our soldiers" but that "because we're so good at all the things we do here...occasionally a patient is tempted to think of us as his personal concierge service. This is a mistake." B.D. responds, "I can tell." Jewel says, "Then let the fun begin! Drain your wound?"

## WHAT WE'RE MISSING:
## REPORTING ON THE SHORTAGE

Although many media pieces about the nursing shortage focus on numbers, some items show why it matters that we don't have enough nurses. Will Moredock's March 2007 cover story on the shortage in the *Charleston City Paper* included an admirably detailed look at what Medical University of South Carolina Hospital ICU nurse Misty Deason actually does for patients. The piece seemed to reflect the writer's surprise at the importance of bedside nursing. Moredock said studies showing that nurse staffing and education levels affect patient outcomes were "startling discoveries." And he seemed to marvel at the credentials of his expert sources, nursing leaders with PhDs — even writing that the name of one source appears on "more than a dozen" publications.

In July 2004 the *New York Times* ran a powerful report by Celia W. Dugger about the catastrophic effects of the emigration of Malawian nurses to developed nations. Dugger outlined the staggering depletion of health resources in AIDS-ravaged Malawi. But her focus was the labor and delivery ward at Lilongwe Central Hospital, where "a single nurse often looks after 50 or more desperately ill people." One nurse found a baby on his mother's breast, desperate to breathe; she reached him in time to suction his tiny mouth until he was able to breathe on his own. The article described the nurse's inability to attend a birth and prevent vaginal tearing, and her later efforts to persuade the fearful, suffering mother to let her suture the tear. One night, after a day nurse had "steadfastly" tried to keep the premature babies in the nursery alive, "a tiny baby girl, blue and dead, lay next to her sister, eyes open, tiny fists clenched, mouth yawning."

A cover story by John Pekkanen in the September 2003 *Reader's Digest* focused on the recent hospital experiences of patients and nurses in the United States. These stories revealed a system on the verge of breakdown, as angry family members struggled to get the attention of overwhelmed nurses and patients died needlessly because there simply weren't enough nurses.

Technology can never fill all the critical roles that nurses play. For instance, every time a nurse enters a patient's room, she observes his or her color, demeanor, state of mind and speech. Any subtle change can signal trouble. [Deceased liver donor] Mike Hurewitz failed to get this sort of assessment — and none of the devices he was hooked up to could perform that job.

Some pieces focusing on the nursing shortage have ably conveyed what public health nurses do. For instance, in February 2004, *Salon* posted a powerful piece by school nurse Elisabeth Ochs, who detailed her efforts to care for about 800 elementary school students. School nurses now care for an increasing number of students suffering chronic conditions like asthma and obesity. In a September 2005 *Salon* article, Laurie Udesky described the "often tragic results" that ensue when unqualified school workers try to give life-saving medications. Kids have died from conditions like asthma and cardiac arrest because there was no school nurse.

## A NURSE DID WHAT?
## PUBLIC HEALTH NURSES IN THE NEWS

Even apart from shortage pieces, the media seems to be somewhat interested in the work of public health nurses. Perhaps the work of these nurses is striking because many don't expect to see nurses improve outcomes using *real skill by themselves.*

The school-nurse-as-one-time hero article has become its own minor genre. In December 2007 the *Dallas Morning News* ran a piece by Chris Coats about a tenacious school nurse who had pushed — in the face of physician skepticism — until an eight-year-old student was correctly diagnosed with leukemia in time to benefit from life-saving treatment. And in October 2006, the Kansas City ABC television affiliate KMBC reported that a local high school nurse had been "credited with saving a student's life" by diagnosing a brain aneurysm.

Other public health nurses have also gained some attention for their work. There have been stories about the Nurse-Family Partnership (NFP), a cost-effective U.S. program in which nurses make prenatal and postnatal home visits to improve the health of poor first-time mothers and their children. A February 2006 issue of *The New Yorker* included Katherine Boo's lengthy "Swamp Nurse," which described the impressive work of rural Louisiana nurse Luwana Marts. The article told how, despite huge obstacles, Marts and her NFP colleagues question, teach, and cajole their patients toward better lives.

## NINETY POUNDS AND THE TRUTH:
## NURSING RESEARCH AND INNOVATION

Some recent press items have highlighted the work of nurses on the cutting edge. In January 2008 the *Manchester Evening News* (UK) reported that nurses at Stepping Hill Hospital had shown that using a particular skin wash greatly reduced the risk of developing the virulent staph infection MRSA from devices like intravenous catheters. A July 2006 article by David Kohn in the *Baltimore Sun* reported that research by nursing scholars showed the burdensome practice of preoperative fasting often confers no benefit. And a January 2006 item by Alan McEwen on the *Scotsman* site described a life-saving initiative by Edinburgh nurse Scott McLean to enable paramedics to treat heart attack victims with "clot-busting" thrombolytic drugs.

Some recent articles have highlighted the trend at urban trauma centers to have specially trained forensic nurses take the lead in caring for sexual assault victims and gathering related evidence. In October 2006 *Newsweek* posted "'CSI' Nursing," a Web exclusive by Anne Underwood introducing readers to forensic nursing. There was also an interview with New Jersey sexual assault forensic examiner (SAFE) nurse Beryl Skog, who explained how she cares for victims and gathers vital evidence for criminal prosecutions.

And although the media generally reserves its career "health care hero" narrative for physicians, nurse researchers have occasionally slipped into the story. In March 2006 Geoffrey Cowley's long *Newsweek* piece about UNAIDS director physician Peter Piot briefly told how, two decades earlier, "ebullient, 90-pound" Kenyan nurse Elizabeth Ngugi pioneered programs that empowered poor Nairobi sex workers to adopt safer sex practices. Ngugi's methods prevent thousands of HIV infections each year. And a March 2004 *Parade* magazine cover story profiled six "superstars" of health research, including Loretta Sweet Jemmott, a professor at the University of Pennsylvania and "the nation's leading expert on HIV prevention in teens."

## "NO ONE WANTS TO HEAR FROM A NURSE": THE NURSE AS MEDIA HEALTH EXPERT

In a November 2006 *ER* episode, nurse character Sam Taggart declined a chance to speak to a local TV news crew about the ED's work because "no one wants to hear from a nurse." This attitude is sadly common among nurses, who often seem determined to keep their heads down, as Buresh and Gordon have shown.

Even so, in November 2006 the *New Zealand Herald* ran a story by Cherie Taylor that relied mainly on "diabetes nurse and educator" Shona Tolley in discussing efforts to address diabetes among the Maori and other indigenous peoples. In May 2006 Rosalind Feldman, RN, DNSc, published a piece in the *Washington Post* describing the poor care she received when she was hospitalized for a femur break, providing a balanced account of the risks of a hospital stay. In a January 2005 column in the *New York Times*, Jane Brody relied heavily on an *American Journal of Nursing* report by Elaine J. Amella, RN, PhD, to address key issues people face as they age. And in September 2004 National Public Radio aired a piece by Patricia Neighmond about the cardiac rehabilitation former President Bill Clinton would undergo following his quadruple bypass surgery; the report included significant expert comment from UCLA cardiac rehab nurse Veronica Polverari.

Some nurses have made it a key part of their careers to provide general health care advice through the mass media. Pat Carroll has given such advice on NBC's *Today Show* and in *Reader's Digest*, and in 2004 she published the helpful book *What Nurses Know and Doctors Don't Have Time to Tell You*. Donna Cardillo has made similar efforts, for instance appearing on NBC's *Weekend Today* in 2003 to discuss the nursing shortage.

## HEY! WHAT ABOUT THESE NURSING ERRORS? OVER HERE!

Few nurses may welcome it, but it is vital that the media train as much attention on nursing errors as it does on physician errors. If nurses want respect for their professional practice, they must also accept responsibility for it. That means helping the public understand that nursing practice problems can mean the difference between life and death.

We're not aware of any recent major report focusing on nursing errors in the comprehensive way physician errors are often discussed. But a few articles have drawn attention to isolated nursing errors where there are sensational bad results. In January 2008 the *Washington Post* ran a piece by Paul Duggan describing a "scathing" report about poor nursing and medical care at St. Elizabeths, a large DC psychiatric hospital. The report found that poor care may have been a key factor in deaths and other bad outcomes at the hospital the previous year. And as discussed in chapter 1, stories in the *Capital Times* (Madison, WI) in November 2006 reported that criminal charges had been filed against OB nurse Julie Thao because of a fatal medication error.

# "IS THIS ALL NURSES DO?" MEDIA CONTEMPT FOR NURSING SKILL

Direct expressions of contempt for nursing skill and expertise remain common in some of the most popular and influential media products of our time.

## Hollywood Tells the World Nursing Is for Losers

*Grey's Anatomy* and *House* have attacked nursing more aggressively than any U.S. television shows in decades, though *Grey's* spin-off *Private Practice* is in the running. *ER* and *Scrubs* are far less likely to disparage nursing skill directly, but they have done so, as have many non-health care shows. So have the recent popular films *Akeelah and the Bee* and *Gracie*.

### GREY'S ANATOMY: "YOU'RE THE PIG WHO CALLED MEREDITH A NURSE"

Though most clinical scenes in *Grey's Anatomy* have no nurses, the few that do generally present nursing as a matter of fetching physicians, or holding or moving things for physicians, usually at the edge of the frame. The few nurse characters who do speak tend to be bitter or fawning lackeys.

The show's March 2005 premiere stressed that smart, tough, attractive women like its surgeon stars do *not* become nurses. In one scene, intern Alex diagnoses a post-op patient as having pneumonia. He tells the older, far less attractive nurse to start antibiotics. The nurse bleats, "Are you sure that's the right diagnosis?"

He responds, "Well, I don't know, I'm only an intern. Here's an idea, why don't you go spend four years in med school and let me know if it's the right diagnosis. She's short of breath, she's got a fever, she's post-op. Start the antibiotics."

Alex tells hot intern Meredith Grey, "God, I hate nurses." Meredith notes that it might not be pneumonia. Alex: "Like I said, I hate nurses." Meredith: "What did you just say? Did you just call me a nurse?" Alex: "Well, if the white cap fits." Meredith stalks off. Later Alex responds to a page from this same nurse, who argues that the patient is still short of breath. He blows her off: "Don't page me again." The pathetic nurse watches him go in silence. Later the chief of surgery endorses Meredith's views. The nurse sensed vaguely that something was wrong, but it took a real professional — Meredith — to do anything about it.

The show's second episode, in April 2005, offered more explicit contempt. Meredith's friend, hotshot intern Cristina, tells Alex, "You're the pig who called Meredith a nurse...I hate you on principle."

The female physicians' reactions to the slurs effectively endorse the assumptions that underlie them. Of course, it would not occur to Meredith or Cristina to say anything in defense of nurses. What they care most about is that they not be regarded as nurses themselves.

*Grey's* has mostly backed off on the explicit contempt, but it has continued to present nurses as lost in the face of serious care problems, and nursing as disgusting work that the interns get as a punishment. In a November 2005 episode, Cristina dismissed a nurse from a patient's room, saying that the physicians would let her know if a bedpan needed changing. Rather than responding directly, the nurse paged Cristina to do a series of grotesque bodily fluid tasks. This plotline was likely intended to help nurses. But it suggested that the problem with anti-nurse slurs is not that they're inaccurate: the problem is, as the chief resident noted, that it's "stupid" to "piss off the nurses"—the petty, vindictive cleanup crew of health care. A November 2006 plotline likewise used the "nurse's job" of "digging through crap" as a symbol of professional disaster. Cristina's chief resident punished her by making her sift through the stool of a boy who had swallowed Monopoly pieces. Later the boy started vomiting. Nurse Tyler paged Cristina, who quickly diagnosed a perforated bowel and directed the clueless Tyler to page the chief resident. And a January 2007 episode portrayed attending physician Mark Sloane inflicting seemingly grotesque, trivial nursing tasks on interns Meredith and Alex as a punishment. As always, there was no hint that the tasks might be important to patient outcomes.

*Grey's Anatomy* has made efforts to address concerns that it portrays nurses as unskilled drones, but these have been isolated and deeply flawed. An April 2005 *Grey's* included a formidable dying woman whom Meredith's surgeon mother described as "an excellent nurse." In a September 2006 *Grey's*, nurse Tyler smugly reported that he was part of a team that saved someone's life. In the January 2007 *Grey's* in which Sloane inflicted icky nursing tasks on the interns, the attending also praised nurses as "smart," "helpful," and "already good at their jobs." And late 2007 episodes of *Grey's* introduced operating room (OR) nurse Rose, temporary love interest of star neurosurgeon Derek "McDreamy" Shepherd. Rose was actually capable of light banter *and* basic OR computer repair, an achievement that the show promoted as helping McDreamy "save a life." And Rose's computer skill was the result of a course she took at *college*.

Sadly, none of these plotlines showed how nurses improve outcomes as part of their normal work. A January 2006 *Grey's* episode with a minor plotline about a nursing strike had a few good lines about short-staffing, but on the whole it suggested that the lack of nurses mostly created burdens in administration and trivial bedside matters. A few testimonials that nurses are "smart" or "excellent" mean little when the show has spent years saying the opposite at every turn. As for Rose, she was never more than a lightweight assistant to the surgeons. Derek noted that the college she attended was a "party school," and her computer work actually underlined how baffled the show is by the idea of nursing. If nurses do save lives, it must be when they happen to have some *other* useful skill. The May 2008 season finale had Rose telling Derek she preferred his talking about "boring science stuff" to brooding about a clinical trial — plainly science is a bewildering subject for those little nurses. Rose was a doe-eyed also-ran for McDreamy's affections compared to the "extraordinary" Meredith Grey. After McDreamy went back to Meredith, a September 2008 episode showed the upset Rose accidentally cut McDreamy's hand with a scalpel, then flee in embarrassment to a job in pediatrics.

## *HOUSE:* "I DON'T USE NURSES"

As on *Grey's*, *House* nurses may appear occasionally to perform basic tasks, like moving a gurney. But *House* nurses are even less likely to appear, and when they do they are even more likely to be silent, peripheral clerks who scurry out of the way of physicians and even patients, to whom they never speak. And whereas the direct attacks on nursing in *Grey's* have mostly been delivered by pretty young physicians, on

*House* they are usually delivered by the brilliant lead character, who sees nurses as unskilled morons. None of House's slurs has been disproved, so viewers mistakenly conclude that the slurs may be mean, but they are as ruthlessly correct as his other diagnoses.

One notable May 2005 episode told how House lost partial use of his leg to muscle cell death after a clotted aneurysm led to an infarction. At one point House was in his ICU bed recovering from an operation to restore circulation in his leg. The monitor showed wide-complex tachycardia. House impatiently told the nurse to give him more calcium gluconate. The nurse responded that he had just gotten 5 ml. He insisted. Nurse: "I'll talk to your doctor." House told her that would take too long, as he had a wide-complex tachycardia and would soon go into cardiac arrest. Her response: "I could get in trouble." House, exasperated and about to lose consciousness, informed the nurse that he was not asking for a narcotic and would soon pass out. He did pass out, and attending physician Lisa Cuddy rushed in, asking the nurse what happened. The nurse said that House had wide-complex tachycardia. "Who diagnosed it?" Cuddy asked. House did, the nurse responded. The nurse handed Cuddy the defibrillation paddles, which Cuddy used.

In less than one minute of screen time, the episode did an amazing amount of damage. First, any ICU nurse would have immediately seen from the monitor that House had wide-complex tachycardia. Yet House had to insist that he was having that problem, and Cuddy's question as to who diagnosed the tachycardia assumed it could not have been the nurse. A real ICU nurse would have told House he needed more calcium gluconate, called the code team, defibrillated, and initiated CPR. House's remark about drug seeking wrongly suggests that nurses are unaware that calcium gluconate is not a narcotic. Without knowledge, initiative, or concern for her patient, all the *House* nurse can do is await the arrival of the almighty Cuddy.

More recently, the House character has made more direct comments on nursing. In November 2005 episodes, House and his assistant physicians suggested that they consider nurses unskilled cleanup staff, good for handling stool and patients who have fallen down. In one priceless scene, House, having just temporarily relieved a patient's thymoma symptoms with a Tensilon injection, went off on a "playing God" riff. When the drug wore off, as expected, the patient fell to the floor. "This," said House, "was exactly why I created nurses;" then he called out into the hallway, "Cleanup on aisle three!"

In a November 2006 episode, physician Foreman prepared to take a sample of spinal fluid from a patient. When the patient's eleven-year-old sister offered to help, Foreman agreed, noting that it's "quicker than calling a nurse." When Foreman instructed the girl to hold her brother's legs still, she asked, "Is this all nurses do?" Foreman responded, with a wry smile, "My boss [House] doesn't trust 'em to do anything else."

Like *Grey's*, *House* has run a minor plotline about a nursing strike. In the April 2008 episode, the only effect of the strike seemed to be an overcrowded ED, revealed in a scene that implied the physicians just had to work harder — as if they could do everything nurses do. As House glibly said, he does not "use nurses" and does not even know what they do. Viewers did briefly see the wife of the episode's main patient/puzzle — a nurse — diagnose her husband's heart attack and save his life by performing CPR. But aside from that, the nurse was as clueless about technical care as the show's wallpaper nurses.

And in a May 2008 episode, after House sustained a head injury, the show had a home health nurse test his pupils with a penlight while he slept. House woke, and the nurse introduced herself as

Nurse Dickerson. House: "I don't need your name. And I got your profession from your supercompetent technique of melting my retinas."

## OTHER HOLLYWOOD TELEVISION SHOWS

Many other shows have also presented nurses as unskilled. Nurses make easy targets for insults and jokes, because writers can count on much of the audience's sharing a sense of nursing as a silly job involving dim females and bodily functions.

Fall 2007 episodes of *Private Practice* introduced the show's LA "wellness clinic," with cute surfing receptionist Dell Parker, a nurse studying to be a midwife. Despite his good intentions, Dell seemed to be the least knowledgeable major nurse character in the last decade of prime-time U.S. television. Dell occasionally helped the clinic physicians as a layperson might. One episode had the physicians teach him how to do Pap smears, though the show also laughed at his babbling about giving a "happy Pap." But why would any nurse work as a receptionist, instead of getting nursing experience and making two to four times as much money? Evidently the show sees little real difference between a nurse and a receptionist. (Maybe this is what "RN" stands for in Hollywood: Receptionist Nurse.)

*ER* has also denigrated nursing skill and professional status. In one September 2006 episode, new physician Abby Lockhart was the mother of a premature infant in the NICU. The two NICU nurses with speaking parts were utterly incompetent. One was a lactation consultant. Though Lockhart was plainly troubled, this nurse was oblivious. She tried to get Lockhart to breastfeed, proclaiming that "breast is best!" and advising that the breast shield goes "between the boob and the tube!" This platitudinous fool did not come off as someone with a college education. The episode also functioned as an attack on breastfeeding advocates, many of whom are nurses. The other NICU nurse blithely dismissed the concerns of Lockhart's mother about a critical heart monitor alarm. Mom had to virtually yell at the nurse to get the physicians — the real life savers. The infant was rushed to surgery. *ER* has shown physician incompetence, but it's rarely if ever this extreme, and there are always plenty of counterexamples.

A May 2004 *ER* episode illustrated the show's traditional view that smart nurses excel by going to medical school. In the episode, then-nurse Lockhart passed her medical boards, a fitting end to a season in which the show exhaustively chronicled her medical school experiences, while (as usual) ignoring the professional development of nurses. No one suggested that Lockhart's move would be a loss to nursing. In fact, though *ER* also had its 1990s major nurse character Carol Hathaway flirt with medical school, nurses are one hundred times more likely to attend graduate school in nursing than in medicine. But the show never presented that as an option for its nurse characters until — after we had been making these points for years — October 2008 episodes indicated that Sam Taggart was starting a nurse anesthetist program. But the show has repeatedly had its characters (particularly nurses) celebrate what it sees as Lockhart's elevation to physician status and, in a May 2008 episode, even celebrate her new attending physician status.

That May 2004 *ER* episode also included an example of the virulent anti-nurse comments that authoritative physician characters have made. After Taggart asked Lockhart if she could cover a nursing shift, attending Kerry Weaver snapped, "Find another nurse. [We] can't have one of our interns changing bedpans during their residency." The nurses had no significant reaction. Weaver was not just saying Lockhart did not have time; she was saying nursing was now beneath Lockhart. Abrasive characters on *ER, House,* and *Grey's* have often made similarly scathing statements about nursing. When the shows fail to offer any rebuttal, they send the message that the comments may be harsh, but they are the unvarnished truth.

*Scrubs* has also suggested that nursing is really low-skilled assistive work. In a notable February 2007 episode, chief of medicine Bob Kelso simply took over as "head nurse" while Carla Espinosa was on maternity leave. Kelso's foray into "nursing" included silly girl talk, trivial scheduling tasks, and references to giving "meds."

---

### I WAS A LOSER AT THE MOVIES

In some recent Hollywood films, nursing has been a dead-end job that the sad women of yesteryear may have had to settle for instead of medicine. But today girls can actually achieve something worthwhile in work and in life.

Yay.

Doug Atchison's *Akeelah and the Bee* (2006) tells the story of an eleven-year-old girl from a struggling Los Angeles school who aims for the National Spelling Bee. Akeelah's widowed mother, Tanya, is barely keeping it together raising the family by herself. Fair enough, except that the film tells us that the bitter Tanya had to settle for being a nurse instead of a physician after dropping out of college. In other words, nurses are sad physician wannabes who lack college-level training.

Davis Guggenheim's *Gracie* (2007) takes a similar approach. In the earnest 1970's era sports drama, a New Jersey student is determined to honor the memory of her dead brother by taking his place on their high school soccer team. But she faces obstacles including a chauvinist father who won't coach her, mocking peers, and a resistant school. The film uses Gracie's angry mother, a nurse who wanted to be a physician, to show that past generations of ambitious women were stuck in dead-end jobs.

---

To mock nurse Kelso, attending Perry Cox ordered him to get Cox some fresh scrubs from housekeeping. Of course, the idea that Kelso could step directly into any nurse's job is absurd. A February 2005 episode focused on what happens to the hospital staff during a quarantine. At one point Espinosa told her surgeon husband Turk that "we're shorthanded" and asked him to redress a patient's bedsores. Turk said "that's nurse stuff" and he did not "have the expertise." Espinosa responded that "any idiot can be a nurse." Turk: "I know." Espinosa shoved him, saying, "I knew you thought that. I knew it." We see that Espinosa objects to Turk's rudeness, but that does not disprove what he said.

Popular shows that do not focus on health care are still prone to disdainful references to nursing skill. In fall 2006 episodes of NBC's drama *Heroes,* hospice nurse Peter Petrelli was one of the "ordinary" people who revealed special powers that would help them *save the world*. Despite a couple of generic references to nursing skill, the series premiere presented hospice nursing as a dead-end job for dreamy, unduly self-sacrificing losers, stressing the contempt of Peter's successful family, who saw the work as just sitting with the dying. In the third episode Peter dropped nursing like it was a hot minimum-wage temp job. In a May 2004 episode of ABC's sitcom *8 Simple Rules*, hospital nurse Cate tried to extricate herself from a meeting with a school principal. When she said patients would die if she was not at work, the principal gave her a skeptical look. Cate admitted patients would not die, but said they might wet the bed.

## "More Than a Nurse":
## How the News Media Disrespects Nurses

Even the most respected news media sources belittle nursing. In October 2006 the *Boston Globe* website posted a poll in its business section after a successful nurses' strike at a local hospital. The item said that the strike was about a plan to reduce what were, according to the hospital, "excessively generous" contracts under which the "average nurse...working a 40-hour week makes $107,000 a year." The site then asked if the nurses "deserve this six-figure salary for what they do." The clear suggestion was that they do not. We doubt the paper would have run such a poll about a "six-figure salary" for lawyers, ad executives, or newspaper editors. But for nurses to make such a salary evidently suggests that our society has its priorities all wrong.

In November 2005, National Public Radio's *Morning Edition* ran a report by science correspondent Brenda Wilson about developing world physicians migrating to wealthier nations. At one point Wilson, reporting from a community health center in a Kenyan village, says that "because there are not enough doctors, the center is run by a clinical officer." To explain the expertise of these officers, Wilson says they are "not quite a doctor but more than a nurse." This makes as much sense as saying that someone is not quite a doctor but more than a science correspondent. Nursing has a unique, holistic approach to care, and nurses have a great deal of expertise that physicians do not have.

Also in November 2005, *Good Housekeeping* included seventy-five "surprising" health tips from "doctors" nationwide. Not one tip came from a nurse. But Michael Roizen, MD, of the Cleveland Clinic, did advise readers to improve their hospital care by "supplying the staff with treats." Dr. X offered hot ED tips, like telling patients to lie to the triage nurse about when symptoms began — never to say it was more than four hours earlier — in order to be seen faster. But, he advised, "tell the doctor exactly when symptoms began." Effective triage requires accurate information, which can mean the difference between life and death. And saying that symptoms began more recently will not necessarily get you seen faster.

In February 2007, one *New York Times* Crossword Puzzle included the following as one of its clues: "I.C.U. helpers." The "correct" answer was "RNS." *Helpers*? The reference may seem trivial, but when the premier crossword in the world says that the nurses who play the central role in high-tech ICU care are just peripheral bit players, it has a real effect. And it shows just how ubiquitous the stereotypes are.

Another notable, if subtle, facet of the news media's lack of regard for nursing is its tendency to suggest that nurses who are not actually providing direct care at the bedside are not nursing—indeed, that they are no longer nurses. In other words, nursing is not a science profession that confers enduring status, or that one might pursue through health management, research, advocacy, or policy-making. In April 2006 the *Long Beach Press Telegram* ran a piece about local nurse Judy Fix, who had saved the life of an injured motorist at the roadside. The headline: "Ex-Nurse Didn't Forget." Fix was referred to as an "administrator" at Memorial Medical Center and a "former nurse." In fact, Judy Fix was the hospital's chief nursing officer and senior vice president of patient care services, managing 1,800 RNs. The media would not refer to Memorial's chief of medicine as an "ex-physician." No one ever called political leaders Bill Frist or Howard Dean "former" physicians. What's the difference? The view that nursing involves simple physical labor and not professional expertise.

## "Don't Forget to Pack a Nurse": Even Good Intentions Can Go Wrong

In recent years many media items have tried to pay tribute to nurses. Unfortunately, even these efforts can suggest that nurses are not so much skilled professionals as they are noble, hardworking, and useful in the way a tool is.

The *New York Times* has run headlines comparing nurses to inanimate health care equipment. In a basically helpful November 2002 "Cases" piece in the *Times,* physician Abigail Zuger suggested that an elderly patient of hers who had died might have survived if not for the nursing shortage. The headline was "Prescription, Quite Simply, Was a Nurse." In September 2005 the *Times* ran a piece by Alina Tugend in its Business section about the trend toward hiring private nurses to compensate for hospital short-staffing. The headline: "Going to the Hospital? Don't Forget to Pack a Nurse."

Tributes to nurses often focus on their willingness to endure hardship. In a May 2005 edition of the *Mercury* (South Africa), Xoliswa Zulu's "Have You Thanked a Nurse Today?" marveled at nurses' endurance and ability to tolerate foul-smelling wounds and bedpans. Readers did not get a sense that nurses are educated professionals.

At times nurses and their supporters seem to embrace this way of thinking. Prominent recent campaigns aimed at addressing the nursing shortage have included the television component of Johnson & Johnson's Campaign for Nursing's Future, which developed three ad campaigns, one each in 2002, 2005, and 2007; travel nurse company Access Nurses' 2006 Internet-based reality show *13 Weeks*; and the University of Michigan's 2007 radio ads featuring men describing why they became nurses at "U of M." All the campaigns presented nurses as good people who work hard to make a difference. But aside from the *2007* J&J television ads, none gave much sense of nursing skill or expertise, and none stressed that nurses improve outcomes. Instead, the focus was on touching, caring, helping, and inspiring.

# IF IT'S IMPORTANT WORK, CREDIT ANYONE BUT A NURSE

In many entertainment and news media products, nursing work is seen to have real value. It saves patients' lives and improves outcomes. That would be great — except that the work is presented as having been done by someone else.

## Physician Nursing: Prime-Time Physicians Do Nursing Work

Every popular hospital show features rampant physician nursing: the shows' structure makes it inevitable. Virtually every major character is a physician, and prevailing practice is that the drama must run through these characters. But because the real physician role is actually somewhat limited, physician characters are often shown doing dramatic work in which real-life nurses take the lead, including bedside monitoring and interventions, psychosocial care, patient advocacy, and education.

*Grey's Anatomy* may have more physician nursing than any other current Hollywood drama. In one May 2008 episode, cardiac surgeon Erica Hahn provided emotional care to a distraught transplant candidate in isolation. Resident Alex Karev gave the patient IV medication. When the patient's lung collapsed, Karev alone intervened to save her, issuing a command to the ether to get Hahn. A nurse-blur responded, "Right away, Dr. Karev!" Resident Meredith Grey provided all psychosocial care to a soldier with a brain tumor. She managed the tension between this soldier's father and his male lover. After the surgery, Meredith monitored the patient's intracranial pressure. Later the patient coded, and a nurse handed Meredith the paddles so she could defibrillate. In real life, every one of these actions would be performed primarily or completely by a nurse.

Karev even got the transplant patient's family into protective gear so they could enter the isolation bubble with her. A nurse would actually have done that, and much sooner. Finally, resident Cristina Yang gave a bitter speech about another surgeon's winning a medical award without crediting her help. She complained — without irony — that she was "the unseen hand to his brilliance," an astonishing echo of the episode's own crediting of physicians for work nurses really do.

In a December 2005 *Grey's* episode, nine hours after a quintuplet birth, each of the five major intern characters sat in the NICU keeping watch over his or her own quint, with no nurses in sight. Of course, nurses monitor real NICU patients; no intern would have a leading role in NICU monitoring or care. The physician characters also provided co-bedding for the quints and emotional support for the quints' distressed mother. The nurses who did appear almost never addressed patients. Perhaps that would be presumptuous with physicians in the room! The same episode also suggested that physicians have all responsibility for patient outcomes. One subplot involved a patient Alex "killed" when he "told a nurse" to administer an incorrect dosage of hypertonic saline, thus dehydrating the patient's brain. No one suggested that the nurse (Olivia) had a duty to scrutinize unfamiliar care plans, which Alex's clearly was.

In an April 2005 *Grey's* episode, intern Izzie tried to help a slightly wounded, resistant older ED patient from China. Unable to find a translator, Izzie gave up, but when she saw the woman leaving, she followed her outside to the rainy parking lot. There was a more seriously wounded younger woman, presumably her daughter. They refused to come inside because the daughter was undocumented, so Izzie stitched and bandaged the daughter's head wound by herself in the rain. In real life, nurses would have provided much of this care, negotiating the cultural barriers, advocating for an experienced surgeon, and providing discharge planning and education.

As we've seen, *House* also generally has physicians do everything important in the hospital. House's team does the work of many health workers besides nurses, including physicians with other specialties. In a May 2006 episode, the physicians did virtually all monitoring, psychosocial care, and therapeutic care. The most amusing part was a nurse-free scene in which physician Robert Chase walked a patient with major facial swelling around after his surgery and even took him to the toilet. Perhaps a physician has done this, but we've never heard of it. And in the May 2008 *House* season finale, when a patient had multiple organ failure, the physician team did the usual range of critical nursing tasks. They infused solutions and IV medications. They set up and maintained a cardiac bypass without nurses. They did ambu-bagging, which nurses or respiratory therapists usually do. They provided all monitoring and psychosocial care. They performed nurse-free surgeries. They induced hypothermia with cooling blankets. They alone performed resuscitation and effected an inter-hospital transfer of the critical patient. None of these things would happen without nurses.

On *ER,* where nurse characters have far more realistic roles than their counterparts on other dramas, there is still plenty of physician nursing. And just as on the other shows, mute nurses provide the dramatic wallpaper for many trauma scenes.

In a May 2007 *ER* episode, nurse Taggart generally came off as a tough, skilled patient advocate, but the care of a physicist with septic shock featured relentless physician nursing. In the ED, Taggart called for the hospital's rapid response team to help this unstable patient. The team was composed solely of physicians and med students. In fact, rapid response teams generally consist mainly of nurses. A wallpaper nurse helped OR resident Neela Rasgotra push the physicist's gurney from the surgical ward to the ICU. But the nurse did not seem to be managing the second-to-second care of oxygenation, IV drips, and cardiovascular stability, as real nurses do during these trips. When ICU attending Kevin Moretti approached, the nurse departed without a word — and without conducting the usual comprehensive verbal and physical handoff to the ICU nurse. The patient crashed, and while Moretti, Rasgotra, and a med student resuscitated her, a bit of a nurse did appear at the edge of the frame a couple of times. The episode also included an intern taking a patient to CT scan alone, a serious ambulance admit with no nurse involvement, and physician medication administration.

A November 2006 *ER* plotline illustrated the show's continuing refusal to admit that SAFE nurses, not physicians, typically take the lead in sexual assault care at major trauma centers. This plotline involved Danielle, a school girl. Attending Luka Kovac saw that Danielle appeared to have been sexually assaulted. He asked physician Lockhart to do the rape exam. Veteran ED nurse Haleh Adams set up the exam materials for Lockhart. As Lockhart gently explained the procedure to the frightened Danielle, Adams stood by silently. Later Lockhart reported to Kovac and a police officer that the rape exam evidence was ready. When surgical resident Neela Rasgotra came to examine Danielle's cuts, Danielle suggested to Rasgotra that the cuts were not too deep, implying they were self-inflicted. Rasgotra asked how she knew the cuts were not deep. Adams finally found her voice, asking gently, "Honey…did you do this to yourself?" It turned out that she had, apparently as a result of witnessing a brutal rape of her mother long ago. In this powerful story, nurses were passive bit players, instead of the clinical leaders they really are.

Physician nursing infects non-hospital shows as well. In the August 2005 series finale of HBO's *Six Feet Under,* major character Brenda went into premature labor. Nurses seemed to be part of the delivery, but they said nothing. One nurse silently transferred the newborn from the obstetrician who delivered it to the warmer, but only the physician spoke, offering limited guidance and reassurance to Brenda. In the post-partum and NICU scenes, no nurse appeared. Instead, a neonatologist tried to provide the distressed Brenda with some support and information. Physicians were portrayed as saving her baby, and Brenda thanked the neonatologist.

And a November 2004 episode of NBC's *Law and Order: Special Victims Unit* featured a special spin on physician nursing. In the episode, commendably, a "sexual assault nurse" character actually examined a rape victim. Sadly, the show depicted one of its two main *detective* characters directing and doing the key work. In real life, the forensic nurse would have directed and provided all the critical care and forensic work, and the police probably would not even have been present. But here, the nurse character came off as an awkward and insensitive assistant, as the detective explained what was going on, took photos, and provided the only real emotional support the patient received.

## Physician Nursing: The Press Misinforms Its Readers

### PHYSICIANS GET THE CREDIT

Many news accounts, particularly those written by physicians, literally assign credit for nursing work to physicians. In May 2007 the *New York Times* ran a long piece by reporter Lawrence K. Altman, MD, about New Jersey Governor Jon Corzine's recovery from a serious auto crash: "In Corzine's Recovery, Doctors Cite Grit and Luck." The article implied that physicians provided virtually all of

Corzine's bedside care. He spent eighteen days in Cooper University Hospital, eleven in the ICU — where elite nurses take the lead 24/7, running high-tech machinery, managing a complex regimen of medications and other treatments, and monitoring patients for the slightest changes in condition. Yet in the midst of many statements about what physicians thought and did, the only specific credit any nurse got in this article was for lip-reading Corzine's requests for medication and water while he was on the ventilator. Altman wrote that Dr. Michael E. Goldberg was "the anesthesiologist who controlled" Corzine's pain medication. Presumably this physician wrote prescriptions and checked in, but nurses monitored Corzine's pain 24/7 and controlled it. Nurses monitor patients for level of consciousness, heart rate, blood pressure, skin color and moisture, grimacing, and other signs of pain on a minute-to-minute basis to titrate the medicine. The article noted, "At Cooper, doctors typically take turns caring for trauma patients every day." The writer must have meant that different physicians are assigned to such patients on different days, but for most readers, this statement would likely confirm the prevailing misconception: physicians do all the important "caring" at the bedside for critical patients like Corzine.

Later that same month, the U.S. Department of Transportation sponsored a public service announcement (PSA) featuring Gov. Corzine urging television viewers to use seat belts. Corzine credited "a remarkable team of doctors and a series of miracles" with saving his life. The PSA was a good public health effort, but it ignored the nurses and other "team" members who likely provided most of the skilled care that saved his life.

In August 2007 the *Times* ran a "Cases" item in which physician Larry Zaroff described how he had helped to save the life of a cardiac patient in 1961. Zaroff arrived to find a nurse and respiratory therapist "desperately trying to keep the patient alive." Then, when the defibrillator "arrived," "current flowed through the patient," a statement that is curiously vague about who actually did the defibrillating. But when Zaroff told of meeting the patient later in the context of a dispute, the vagueness was gone. Zaroff told the patient, "I was the one who saved your life, brought your heart back." The team effort had become the work of the physician alone.

In October 2004 a long, unsigned article in the *Wall Street Journal* on allowing family presence during major hospital procedures recognized that nurses had been most active on that issue and even featured quotes from nursing experts. Unfortunately, even that article repeatedly suggested that physicians alone perform the major procedures and that the nurses are largely observers who have time to worry about how the family may react. The first sentence referred to steps to alleviate "one of medicine's most trying ordeals: That wait in the hall while doctors are working on a loved one." Later, the piece noted that a Boston hospital had begun allowing family members to stay during codes when "doctors may need to shock the patient or open up the chest to massage the heart." And one of the reported benefits of family presence? "Families can give on-the-spot medical information to trauma doctors."

## PHYSICIANS GET THE BLAME

The media commonly assigns all blame for health care errors and problems to physicians, often in the context of malpractice articles. It would be natural for nurses and other health workers not to object. But they should, because this practice signals that the media and society regard physicians as the ones who provide all important care, including much that nurses really do. Being seen as an integral part of the health care picture means receiving due credit when things go well, and due responsibility when things do not.

A September 2008 *New York Times* article by Laurie Tarkan discussed emergency patients' poor understanding of their care. Patient education is a key nursing responsibility, and nurses generally spend far more time on it than physicians do, at least if staffing allows. But this piece gave no hint of that fact, instead relying on multiple statements from five named physicians. Not one nurse was consulted, though nurses did get a mention—in discussion of a "dual discharge" approach in which a physician discusses care with patients and a nurse "follows up with computerized discharge instructions."

In June 2004 the *Times* published a column by Bob Herbert about two malpractice claims against an ob/gyn. In the first case, the piece suggested that a critical problem for a baby born with "severe brain damage" was improper checking of a fetal monitoring strip while the physician was absent. Herbert stated, with unmistakable contempt, that the physician "blamed the ensuing tragedy on the nurse." In fact, the apparent monitoring and assessment error described *would* generally be a nurse's job. If this nurse was unqualified, the problem remains a nursing problem. The other case Herbert cited involved serious intestinal damage caused to a patient who had a sponge left inside her during a cesarean section. Certainly, the ob/gyn—who monitored the patient's worsening pain for months of outpatient visits and failed to identify the cause—would seem to be partly responsible. But the nurse attending the C-section had a duty to account for the number of sponges used, to avoid mistakes just like this. There is no hint of that fact in Herbert's account of the case.

Two days later the *Times* ran a piece by Alex Kuczinski and Warren St. John about two plastic surgery deaths at the elite Manhattan Eye, Ear and Throat Hospital. Novelist Olivia Goldsmith had died, apparently of cardiac arrest related to anesthesia received while she was getting a "chin tuck." The writers said a nurse anesthetist gave Ms. Goldsmith anesthesia, noting that this is a common practice, perhaps lest anyone wonder whether this in itself was a safety issue. However, the nurse anesthetist was not named, nor was there further discussion of his or her role — even though the piece described the alleged failure to monitor respiration and cardiac activity, for which the nurse anesthetist would presumably have been responsible. But the anesthesiologist involved in the other death was named a number of times, as were the surgeons in both cases. The idea seemed to be that a mere nurse could not be ultimately responsible. Less surprising was the failure to mention the roles of registered nurses, who would presumably have been involved in both surgeries, and whose job is to monitor patient conditions.

In December 2005 the *Baltimore Sun* ran Fred Schulte's massive series "Masking Malpractice Cases." The gist was that Maryland's system for overseeing physician practice was failing to protect patients because of misguided regulatory practice and the overuse of confidentiality. The article focused on the small number of physicians who have had unusually high numbers of malpractice claims or payments. Readers would plainly see the *Sun's* report as addressing the full universe of health care errors. Yet there are four times as many registered nurses as physicians, and although nurses are not seen as the litigation targets physicians are, there is no reason to think nurse errors are any less numerous or consequential. But in this entire *Sun* report, whose text exceeded 9,500 words, neither the word "nurse" nor the word "nursing" appeared even once.

## Nursing Just Happens

Many press pieces effectively suggest that important nursing care has been done by hospitals or machines, or else that it has simply occurred, with no actor named.

In Lawrence Altman's *New York Times* report about Gov. Corzine's recovery, readers learned that Corzine "received 12 pints of blood." And they heard about "the drugs that Mr. Corzine received in intensive care." Nurses give blood and drugs, and it is not simple or easy. "There were potential fatal complications: pneumonia; other infections; acute respiratory distress syndrome; blood clots in the leg that could travel to the lungs or other organs and cause emergencies, if not sudden death." Indeed, avoiding those complications was critical to Corzine's survival. The only thing missing from the article was some indication of which health professionals took the lead in preventing them: nurses. Gov. Corzine's PSA attributed his survival in part to the fact that a "ventilator was breathing for me." But the ventilator did not run itself. Nurses and respiratory therapists carefully monitored Corzine's tolerance to the ventilator, weaned him off it, and taught him how to breathe without it.

Or consider a September 2003 *Times* piece Dr. Altman wrote for the well-named "Doctor's World" feature about the care of U.S. Marines who had gotten severe cases of malaria in Liberia. The piece mostly suggested that physicians did everything of note, worrying about the symptoms, starting injections, inserting breathing tubes. But at certain points, when nurses almost certainly played a key role, more general terms were used: the sick Marines were greeted by "a medical team" in full protective gear, the "military medical team" examined and cared for them, "the hospital" cleared out a ward to isolate them. Alternatively, the passive voice was employed, so that things were not done by any particular human, they simply occurred. Thus, the Marines "were allowed visitors."

In February 2006 National Public Radio's *Morning Edition* ran a report by Richard Knox about the lack of intensive care resources that would be needed to handle a bird flu pandemic: U.S. hospitals would not have enough ventilators or "hospital beds." The report wrongly implied that care for patients would revolve mainly around whether physicians granted access to the vents or beds, and it quoted only physicians — as if either physicians provide all the associated care, or the vents and hospital beds do it themselves.

## Innovation: Which Non-Nurse Thought of That?

Some recent reports discuss the work nurses do on innovative health projects, often outside the usual clinical settings. But even these pieces may present the nurses as carrying out work engineered by others. Of course, it may be that a specific project *was* designed by someone else. But nurses are not empty vessels into which others have poured expertise. Nurses have long been expert in community health and holistic preventative care, as explained in chapter 1. It often seems that the nursing care model gains attention only when it is embraced by physicians or others with more social status.

Consider recent reports on the work of the Nurse Family Partnership (NFP) to improve the health of poor mothers and children, such as Katherine Boo's February 2006 *New Yorker* article and an August 2007 *CBS Evening News* report by Katie Couric. We have seen no major mainstream article that cites the NFP program's debt to the long tradition of home-based nursing care, so the whole idea that "nurse-visitors" can improve maternal-child health may seem to have originated with NFP founder David Olds, a developmental psychologist. The pieces have also failed to convey how much the nurses' success is due to their nursing skill, not just to Olds's program design or the nurses' personal attributes, trusted image, or on-the-job experience.

In October 2006 an Associated Press piece by Alicia Chang reported that insurers increasingly rely on "health coaches" to help patients manage chronic conditions at home, thereby cutting costs and improving outcomes. The report barely manages to note that most of the coaches are nurses, so it fails to discuss why nurses are uniquely qualified to play such roles. Instead, it credits a Colorado physician for the specific care "model" it discusses, which may imply that this kind of work is a recent physician innovation.

## GHOSTS IN THE MACHINE: NURSES GO MISSING IN THE MEDIA

The media often simply ignores nursing, even when reporting on skilled work in which nurses play a central role, such as hospital care. Nurses are not generally recognized as career health care "heroes," and they are rarely consulted as health experts.

### Lost in Hollywood

Popular Hollywood products often ignore the role nursing would really play in their area of interest. For example, *House* includes many clinical scenes in which no nurses appear, even though the patients are in critical condition and would require a great deal of skilled nursing, such as in the nurse-free cardiac bypass scene in the May 2008 episode. Real nurses play a key role even in the physician diagnosis that dominates *House*, collecting information and raising issues with physicians.

Ignoring nursing also results in a failure to portray recent nurse-led advances in care that television producers would almost certainly take great interest in if the developments had originated with physicians. For instance, in hospital dramas, especially *ER,* family members are forever freaking out to see their loved ones in distress, then causing disruption. Physician characters often command nurses to remove the family. We have never seen a nurse character advocate for family to stay, or discuss the trend toward allowing family presence, which nursing research has shown to have real benefits.

In some respects, Hollywood portrayals of newborn care are similarly behind the times. Recent episodes of *ER, Grey's,* and other shows have focused on NICUs, but they have largely failed to reflect recent nurse-led developments in kangaroo care (keeping the infant at its mom's or dad's chest for certain periods), co-bedding for multiples, or breastfeeding. Of course, this problem can also be linked to the fact that virtually all meaningful input into Hollywood dramas comes from physicians, not nurses.

Unfortunately, most documentaries, reality shows, and daytime shows about health care have taken a similar physician-centric approach. Notable examples include Terry Wrong's two multi-part *ABC News* documentaries, *Hopkins 24/7* (2000) and *Hopkins* (2008). The former focused on the famous hospital's senior physician stars, the latter on the residents (because if there's one thing the public needs to hear more about, it's how new physicians are trained). *Hopkins* did give a few minutes to two pediatric transport nurses, but the vast majority of both series suggested that only physicians really matter in hospital care. And in late 2008, a daily syndicated daytime show called *The Doctors* appeared. This *Dr. Phil* spin-off featured four physicians dispensing health advice and opinions, with a focus on cosmetic plastic surgery. Though nurses are expert in patient education, they seemed to have no real role on *The Doctors*.

## Lost in the News

News items often ignore nurses or nursing, even when covering areas in which nurses play a key role. The 2007 *New York Times* article about Governor Corzine's recovery stated that "hospital aides wheeled Mr. Corzine to the basement for CAT scans" looking for evidence of a variety of serious problems. In fact, coordinating the transfer of such a critically ill patient to and from CT scan is one of the most challenging aspects of ICU nursing. Nurses kept Mr. Corzine alive during that journey, but the *Times* ignored them.

In a June 2004 "Cases" item in the *Times*, Richard A. Friedman, MD, discussed whether July is a perilous time to visit U.S. hospitals because of the influx of recent medical school graduates with little experience. Friedman admitted that it was rational to be concerned about "July syndrome" but argued that there is little basis to think care suffers, because of "vigilant supervision" by attending physicians. In fact, a great deal of the "vigilance" is supplied by nurses, who also play a key role in teaching the interns how to practice safely. But the word *nurse* did not appear in this piece.

When nurses spearhead groundbreaking research or policy proposals, elite media sources often ignore it. In October 2004 the Columbia University School of Nursing issued a press release about its striking plan, published in *Nursing Economics*, to provide universal health coverage in the United States at an annual cost of about $2,000 per person. Despite the obvious link to the impending election, more than a week later the only major press coverage appeared to be a short item by Laura Gilchrest on the *CBS Marketwatch* website. It is hard to avoid the conclusion that the Columbia plan was ignored because of the professional status of those who created and published it. Maybe the mental reaction of editors and reporters went something like this: "What's this? Universal coverage for $2K? Wow! Who's behind this? Oh...what else have we got?"

## Nurses Evacuated from Disaster Areas

It's striking how invisible nursing is in news accounts about responses to mass casualty events, considering the central role nurses would actually play. In early 2007 NPR's *Morning Edition* aired interviews with disaster health experts. In February it ran an interview with a former U.S. Coast Guard officer, who said at one point that a community had to ask whether it could handle hundreds of thousands of casualties, "all requiring triage and other kinds of life-and-death care." Show host Steve Inskeep asked if that meant asking whether such a place had "hundreds of vacant beds...hundreds of idle doctors?" In a March interview, when the chief of medical affairs at a New Orleans hospital noted that a lack of "health care providers" was hampering efforts to restore area hospitals to full capacity after Hurricane Katrina, Inskeep wondered whether even hospitals that had remained open "don't have enough doctors available." In both stories, the experts sooner or later worked nurses into the conversation. In fact, most of the critical care in such emergencies, such as triage, is provided by nurses.

In September 2005 many press sources ran an Associated Press piece by Marilynn Marchione about hospital care after Katrina. The *Yahoo!* headline was typical: "Doctors Emerging as Heroes of Katrina." The AP report portrayed physicians as having done virtually everything of note for patients at New Orleans hospitals after the storm. Apart from a passing reference to RNs and EMTs, and one sentence about a Pennsylvania paramedic, the piece was all physicians all the time, with many references to what "doctors" did, and multiple quotes and description of no fewer than eight named physicians and a medical student. Not one nurse was mentioned, though nurses played a central role in keeping patients alive under the extreme conditions during Katrina.

## Can We Be "Heroes"?

The media often salutes the careers of health care "heroes." Nurses are rarely recognized in this way, though they may be honored for saving a life outside of their normal work settings.

In November 2005, *Time* magazine featured a massive report on global health. Slightly more than half of the total report was devoted to profiles of eighteen "heroes" whose "energy and passion are making a difference" in the fight against disease worldwide. Of the fifteen health care professionals profiled, twelve were physicians. Not one "hero" was recognized for her nursing, though a profile of a nutritionist noted that she had a nursing degree. Only one brief mention in the whole report could be considered a tribute to the work of the world's estimated 12 million nurses to stem disease. That was in the concluding essay by rock star Bono.

In July 2004 Discovery Health Channel aired the *Discovery Health Channel Medical Honors*. The star-studded special saluted thirteen "medical heroes" for "bringing awareness to many challenging health and medical issues of our time." The thirteen honorees consisted of eight physicians, a biosciences researcher, a non-profit leader, a political science professor, a health system CEO, and an ad executive. No nurses made the cut, but nurses were represented — by actress Yvette Freeman, who plays nurse Haleh Adams on *ER* and who appeared at the ceremony as a presenter. You go, nurses!

When nurses do appear as "heroes," it's often because they have surprised people by saving a life outside their normal work setting. In April 2007 the *Globe and Mail* and the *Toronto Star* reported that Canadian pediatric nurse Julie Beattie had saved a heart attack victim at a hockey game. Nicole Brodeur's helpful May 2005 *Seattle Times* column recounted how ED nurse Joanne Endres saved a man having a heart attack on a plane flight. The theme of that column, "Flying Solo, Nurse Is Enough," was that the public does not understand what nurses do. Brodeur proved it by quoting a passenger who said of Endres, "She just knew what to do…. And there wasn't even a doctor there!"

## Nurses? Health Care Experts?

The media regularly fails to consult nurses as experts in health care items. Of course, part of the problem is, as Buresh and Gordon stress, that nurses fail to speak up about their work. The vast majority of the "Cases" and "Doctor's World" items in the *New York Times* are written by physicians. We cannot recall ever seeing one by a nurse until September 2008, when nurse (and former English professor) Theresa Brown managed to publish a powerful "Cases" piece about the death of a cancer patient.

One telling indication of how nurses are regarded was the selection of the Google Health Advisory Council, a group of eminent health "experts" formed in 2007 to help the dominant media company consider how to "contribute to the health care industry." The group of more than twenty prominent health figures included thirteen physicians, and many members without any formal health care training. No nurses.

Press pieces on areas of nursing expertise abound — but without any nursing experts as sources. After the February 2006 National

Public Radio report on bird flu that failed to quote any nurse, a comparable *New York Times* story the next month by Donald G. McNeil Jr. likewise quoted only physicians. Perhaps because neither report sought nursing input, neither explained that the nursing care that keeps critically ill patients alive involves much more than ventilators, or asked where we might get the many additional ICU nurses needed to care for ventilated patients. The NPR piece described a physician proposal to ration access to vents in a pandemic. But sadly, it might not be a wise use of nurses' time to provide *any* ventilator-related care to flu patients — their skills would be better used helping those flu patients with a better chance of survival.

In May 2006 a huge *Time* cover story by Nancy Gibbs and Amanda Bower stressed that not even health workers are safe from the health threats posed by...hospitals. The story, "Q: What Scares Doctors? A: Being the Patient," presented an all-physician vision of hospital care, based on expert comment by twelve physicians. It excluded nurses. At one point, the writers wondered who the "sentinels" and "advocates" in hospitals would be now that family physicians have supposedly been excluded from the role. Hint: that's what the nurses who make up the majority of professional hospital staff do, or would do if they had the staffing and other resources.

## CAN ANY HELPFUL PERSON OR THING BE A NURSE?

The media uses the term *nurse* broadly. It often refers to female caregivers as "nurses" no matter how little health training they have. For example, the Hollywood films *The Skeleton Key* (2005) and *The Grudge* (2004) have been widely promoted as having "nurse" characters, but the characters are actually non-nurse caregivers. The media also reinforces abuse of the term *nurse* by makers of health technology and daycare providers. Of course, the verb form of *nurse* has long been used to describe unskilled tending, especially by females. And as we explained in chapter 1, the term *nurse* can accurately be applied to professionals with a range of educational backgrounds.

Even so, the media has some obligation to consider the effects of its use of the term. It might start by making sure that those it calls "nurses" actually *are* nurses. Let's try the nouns first, and maybe we can work our way up to the verbs!

## I, Robot, Will Be Your Nurse

Sometimes the media refers to new health care technology as a "nurse," as in "electronic nurse," "surgical nurse," and "robot nurse." In some cases, developers or marketers call their products "nurse." These products may assist with nursing tasks, but equating machines with college-educated health professionals is unhelpful.

In January 2007 the *Scotsman* ran Angus Howarth's "Robot Nurses Could Be on the Wards in Three Years, Say Scientists." The piece reported on a project by European Union–funded scientists to develop machines to "perform basic tasks" at hospitals. These include cleaning up spills, guiding visitors around, and perhaps distributing medicines and taking temperatures. The article blithely suggested such robots are "nurses," and it proposed other imaginative names, such as "nursebots" and "mechanised 'angels.'"

Similarly, in March 2006 the website of Wis10 (the Columbia, SC, NBC affiliate) posted an item by Chantelle Janelle, "Health Alert: Electronic Nurse." It described a $70 machine used to help real nurses do home health monitoring by asking patients basic questions. Calling such a machine a "nurse" reinforces the view that nurses serve as mechanical conduits between patients and physicians.

The surgical robot Penelope has attracted a lot of media attention. In Marc Santora's January 2005 *New York Times* piece, physician developer Michael Treat stated that his "robot should be able to do everything a nurse can" and suggested that it would some day replace scrub nurses. But OR nurses do many things that require advanced scientific training, including monitoring surgical practice and the patient's condition, intervening in the case of an emergency, and advocating for the patient. Even after Treat commendably seemed to stop making comments like these, the media could not resist doing it for him. In June 2005 the *New York Daily News* ran an article by Robert Schapiro reporting that Penelope had acted "as a surgical nurse" in a routine operation. Despite at least noting that the robot is "not meant to replace" scrub nurses, the piece still suggested that Penelope is doing nurses' jobs by handing instruments to surgeons. Of course, these robots are no more nurses than they are surgeons, but we have yet to hear of a surgical robot being called an "electronic surgeon."

## You Just Haven't Earned It Yet, Baby Nurse

Many in-home newborn nannies market themselves as "baby nurses," regardless of whether they have any health training. The media has repeated this term, even shortening it to "nurse." This practice continues even though some jurisdictions have made "nurse" a restricted title, in order to protect the public from unlicensed practitioners.

In February 2007 Vickie Elmer's item in the "Jobs" section of the *Washington Post* repeatedly referred to the infant caregiver it profiled as a "baby nurse," even though the provider had virtually no health care training. And in November 2005 the *Baltimore Sun* ran a story by Nicole Fuller about "baby nurses" who were helping a woman who recently gave birth to quintuplets. The pieces described these caregivers as "nurses," but they appear to have been infant care providers who at most had taken a CPR class.

As the *Post* later pointed out, there is a historic association between infant caregiving and the word "nurse," as in "nursemaid." But to use "nurse" this way today sends a damaging message about professional nursing and may also pose more direct risks. Indeed, in August 2005 the *New York Daily News* ran a piece about the lack of regulation and awareness of the minimal training "baby nurses" have. The report, by Pete Donohoe and Caitlyn Kelly, stemmed from the case of Noella Allick, who reportedly "confessed to violently shaking and seriously injuring two babies in her care." The article rightly suggested that a key problem is that anyone can call herself a "nurse." New York State later made "nurse" a protected title. But the term "baby nurse" remains common in major U.S. news media.

## I Say You're a Nurse, and the Shortage Is Over

It's not just the media, of course. In hospitals, many people — including some physicians — refer to any female they come across who is not a physician as a "nurse." Such "nurses" may include technicians, medical assistants, nurses' aides, and clerks. Hospitals may see no reason to clarify matters. Some facilities have placed unlicensed assistive personnel into nursing roles. But when a patient asks an apparent "nurse" with only a few weeks' training to explain his condition, and the "nurse" cannot do so, the patient may conclude that nurses as a group are not skilled or educated.

The media reflects and reinforces this tendency to equate "nurse" with "female hospital worker." For instance, in a 2005 episode of the popular *Dr. Phil* television show, the host — a psychologist — repeatedly referred to a nurse's aide as a "nurse." This aide did not say a word (about anything) during the four minutes she was on the show.

No one, including an actual nurse who was another guest, offered any clarification.

And consider the January 2006 CVS drugstore company television ad in which a pharmacist explained that he had spent several hours teaching a patient's husband to administer her twenty different medications. The pharmacist twice stated that the husband was now "a nurse." Modern drug regimens are complex, and the health financing system has left many families with the impossible task of trying to nurse themselves. But this ad wrongly suggested that pharmacists could train nurses, and that training a nurse might take only a few hours.

This sense that anyone can be a nurse goes hand in hand with ideas to resolve the shortage by recruiting those with few other options. In March 2006 the news magazine *Der Spiegel* ran a piece by Guido Kleinhubbert about a new German government program to train prostitutes to become "care workers for the elderly," including "nurses." The piece had lots of quips comparing the trainees' old and new roles, but it failed to define precisely what they were training for. It is possible they were to be nurse's aides.

But more broadly, a number of initiatives and press pieces in recent years do seem to suggest that solutions to the developed world's nursing shortage lie in sex workers, those on public assistance, desperate nurses from poor nations, or foreign physicians who can't pass their physician licensing exams. Excellent nurses may come from any of these categories. But the sense we get from many of these press stories is that these are all good fits because, after all, to be a "nurse" requires little critical thinking, knowledge, or skill.

The press has also reported unquestioningly on plans to address the shortage by aggressive "streamlining" of nursing educational requirements to get more nurses into practice faster. For example, a

June 2005 article by Joel Dresang in the *Milwaukee Journal-Sentinel* approvingly described a large Wisconsin program that included ideas to "streamline" nursing coursework. Ideas that effectively result in less education for nurses are not necessarily in the interests of nurses or their patients. In some sense, such measures may actually change what a "nurse" is.

Simply finding new groups of people to plug the gaping holes in the nursing workforce does nothing to fix the reasons those holes exist in the first place, which include poor working conditions and a lack of real understanding of nursing. Consider the reaction if similar strategies were applied to shortages of other workers who hold lives in their hands. Would the media uncritically report on plans to address a physician shortage by "streamlining" medical school?

# CHAPTER 4

# Yes, Doctor! No, Doctor!

MOST OF SOCIETY REGARDS physicians as the captains of the health care ship and nurses as their helpful crew. In fact, nursing is an autonomous profession, as we explained in chapter 1. Some media products reflect this reality, but many, particularly television shows like *Grey's Anatomy*, reinforce the damaging myth that physicians manage nurses.

Of course, the media has not simply invented the idea that nurses are physician subordinates. Many physicians themselves believe they manage nurses. The May 2008 issue of *California Lawyer* magazine featured a piece by a physician who had attended Stanford, become a lawyer, and worked at a major national law firm. L. Okey Onyejekwe Jr.'s piece describes his residency at Columbia, from 2000 to 2003:

> I was a 25-year-old resident trying to establish authority in an emergency room where many of the nurses and staff had been practicing since before I was born. Despite being the least-experienced, lowest paid, and youngest person in the ER, I was responsible for managing the ER staff and for the health and well-being of numerous patients.

In fact, as a new resident, Onyejekwe was not "responsible for managing the ER staff." He was one member of a team, reporting to a physician manager. The nurses and others reported to their respective managers. Actually, one of nurses' most important professional roles is to act as an independent check on physician care plans to protect patients and ensure good care. Another key nursing role is to educate physicians, especially residents, about how to recognize changes in patient conditions and respond with appropriate treatments. These roles are rarely acknowledged by physicians or the media.

So why would a new physician think it was his job to "manage" veteran health staff? We doubt he had a medical school course entitled The New Physician's Burden: Managing All Other Health Professionals. We assume his thinking was based on professional and cultural assumptions that nurses and other staff are relatively unskilled subordinates—and so physicians do and must manage all of health care. These ideas are deadly. They contribute greatly to health care errors and poor outcomes.

As we noted in chapter 2, a December 2007 Associated Press article reported that OR nurses at one hospital had failed to stop life-threatening surgical errors because they lacked the practical power to do so. In December 2004 the *Times of India* reported that, after a nurse pointed out to a physician that he had failed to place a used syringe in the proper receptacle, offended physicians chose to "start a fight" with the nurses. Police were called in to restore order. Despite nursing autonomy, physicians still have greater social and economic power, so it is often difficult for nurses to resist their plans. Some nurses have better success. In March 2006 the AP cited a police report that the chief of neurosurgery at an Oakland hospital was "arrested after allegedly throwing a drunken fit when a nurse refused to let him operate." And recall our friend Dan Lynch from chapter 1, the nurse who fought successfully to persuade his heart patient's surgeon that a new heart valve had a potentially fatal problem. Nurses are the patient advocates, the last line of defense. If they are viewed as subordinate, they cannot do their jobs effectively.

The "handmaiden" stereotype sets nurses up as assistants to physicians. It fosters poor relations with some patients and physicians, who sense they can abuse nurses with impunity, a major factor in nursing burnout and the nursing shortage. In November 2005 South Africa's *Cape Argus* reported that research in South Africa, the UK, and the United States suggested that nurses experience disproportionately high physical and psychological violence by patients and colleagues, especially physicians. The article noted that 80 percent of nurses surveyed in a recent South African study said that private sector nurses were leaving the profession because of abuse, largely by male physicians. More recently, a 2008 study found that more than half of U.S. nurses had been bullied on the job, with severe effects on their emotional and physical health.

And the handmaiden stereotype affects who pursues nursing careers. Few ambitious people want to take years of rigorous science courses and endure extraordinary workplace burdens just to be assistants to the professionals who receive all the glory.

## ARE YOU SURE NURSES ARE AUTONOMOUS? IT SURE LOOKS LIKE PHYSICIANS CALL ALL THE SHOTS

Well, it sure looks that way on television. That's what we've been heavily conditioned to see. Diagram 1 (see page 108) shows how most of society views the relation of nurses and physicians.

Yet nursing is a self-governing profession and a distinct scientific discipline. Nurses have a unique, holistic patient advocacy focus, a unique scope of practice under law, and a unique body of knowledge, including special expertise in areas such as public health, wound care, and pain management. As members of an autonomous profession, nurses are educated by nursing scholars, typically in nursing science degree programs at colleges. They use textbooks authored by those scholars. Over 40,000 U.S. nurses have PhDs or other doctoral degrees, and more than 375,000 U.S. nurses have at least a master's degree in nursing. These nurses — not physicians — are the theoretical and practical leaders of the nursing profession. The actual relation of the two disciplines in terms of knowledge is shown in diagram 2.

**People think**

that nurses are supervised by physicians and that nurses know only a tiny subset of what physicians know.

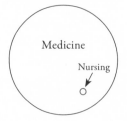

DIAGRAM I

**Who really knows what?**

Nurses and physicians have their own knowledge bases, which overlap. Each has knowledge the other does not.

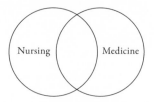

DIAGRAM 2

**Who's really in charge?**

Nurses and physicians are members of separate, autonomous professions. Neither is in charge of the other. They have separate practice acts, codes of ethics, and supervisory and oversight structures. Unfortunately, they are unequal in power, as the different size of these circles reflects.

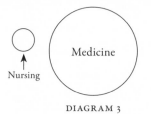

DIAGRAM 3

As diagram 2 illustrates, there is a significant overlap with medicine, but nursing is not a subset of medicine. In the United States, nurse-controlled state boards administer rigorous nurse licensing examinations, and practicing nurses have independent malpractice liability and codes of ethics. State laws typically describe nursing practice in broad terms that do not depend on physicians. California's Nursing Practice Act defines nursing as care that promotes health and requires significant scientific knowledge and skill.[1] It includes patient care, disease prevention, the administration of medications and other procedures "ordered" by physicians or other advanced practitioners, testing procedures, health assessment, and intervention. These state laws make clear that nursing manages itself. And they define nursing practice to include a wide range of critical prevention and care functions that do not depend on physicians or anyone else. Of course, physicians have more practical power. Reasons include the economic benefits physicians receive in health care financing structures, physicians' generally higher levels of education and political clout, long-standing class and gender disparities, and the social esteem physicians enjoy. Diagram 3 shows the basic relation of nursing to medicine in terms of power.

Nurses administer treatments prescribed by advanced practitioners, and some language in these nursing practice acts (e.g., "ordered" in the California law) may suggest a subordinate relationship as to those tasks. In media portrayals, nurses often follow physician "orders" automatically, as if they were mandatory military orders. But nurses have ethical and legal obligations to assess all planned care. Nurses are not relieved of malpractice liability simply because they were administering treatment as prescribed. Nurses' patient advocacy may include persistent negotiation with advanced practitioners, refusing to participate in care plans they deem unsafe, and if necessary getting appropriate authorities to stop such actions.

Do nurses find any of that easy to do, given current power structures? No. Speaking up is especially hard for nurses who have recently immigrated from developing nations to wealthier ones. These nurses may have a tenuous immigration status and families who depend greatly on their continued income. Some may not have been trained to assert themselves with physicians. Does nurses' advocacy sometimes fail because physicians have more power? Of course. Hospitals have fired nurses for advocating for patients, particularly when that advocacy has run counter to the desires of powerful physicians who are seen as revenue generators. Some years ago a Canadian nurse friend was fired from a Caribbean hospital for telling a tourist patient that she should return to the United States for an operation, rather than allow a dangerously inept local surgeon to do it. The physicians pressured nursing managers to fire the nurse. But that still does not make nurses subordinate to physicians.

In fact, nurses have significant practical autonomy in clinical settings. In hospitals, where most U.S. nurses practice, nurses are hired, fired, and managed by other nurses. Hospital nurses are typically led by a chief of nursing, who reports to the hospital's chief executive, not to the chief of medicine. Physicians lack expertise in many areas of nursing, and it would make little sense for them to manage nurses. The same basic structure is found in nursing homes. And in public schools and other public health positions, nurses are effectively autonomous within the scope of their professional duties. Even the nurses who practice in outpatient offices are operating autonomously within the scope of their nursing practice, though they may be employees of a business owned by physicians or others. Nurses must follow their legal and ethical obligations regardless of their employer's identity.

Courts have begun to awaken to the fact that nursing is a distinct scientific profession with its own standards and scope of care. For decades, U.S. courts tended to wrongly regard nursing as a subset of medicine. Accordingly, physicians were permitted to testify as to the standard of nursing care in malpractice actions, as Ellen K. Murphy noted in a November 2004 article in the *Association of periOperative Registered Nurses Journal*. But in *Sullivan v. Edward Hospital* (2004), the Illinois Supreme Court concluded that a physician was not qualified to testify as to a nursing standard of care because he was not a nurse. This case was specific to the Illinois statutory and judicial context, but Murphy rightly described it as "judicial recognition [of] nurses' long-time assertion that nursing is an independent profession with a unique body of knowledge and not simply a subcategory of medicine." In a September 2004 position paper, the American Association of Nurse Attorneys explained why only nurses should be allowed to provide such expert testimony:

> Nursing is a profession, unique, identifiable and autonomous. As a profession, nursing has the authority and responsibility to define its standards of practice....It is clear that the profession of nursing, though closely related to the practice of medicine, is, indeed, distinct with its own licensing scheme, educational requirements, areas of specialization, Code of Ethics, models, theories and contract with society....The nurse is not a "junior doctor" nor is the nurse a mere "underling" of the physician. To so hold would negate the existence of nursing as a profession and would render the Nurse Practice Acts of every state, commonwealth and territory

meaningless. It is unlikely that any physician, unless he/she has completed a nursing program and has practiced as a nurse, can offer competent, reliable expert opinion on these nursing standards.

The notion that nurses report to physicians has several sources. Historically, nurses deferred to physicians, for reasons that include the disparity of power between the genders. And many nurses remain reluctant to challenge physicians or to assert themselves generally, as Bernice Buresh and Suzanne Gordon showed in their groundbreaking book *From Silence to Voice*. More than 90 percent of nurses are still female, and overall gender equality has not been achieved. Assertive women have a wide range of career choices, and many avoid nursing. In addition, physicians' combination of economic power and social status remains unmatched. Physicians have more years of formal education than most (though not all) nurses. Most physicians are not well-informed about nursing, and many believe they are in charge of patient care. Consistent with this authoritarian vision, physician disrespect, disruptive behavior, and even abuse remain issues in many care settings, as Gordon showed in *Nursing Against the Odds* (2005).

Even some nurses and nursing advocates seem to doubt that nursing is autonomous, including Gordon and Dana Beth Weinberg, who wrote *Code Green: Money-Driven Hospitals and the Dismantling of Nursing* (2003). In reaching flawed conclusions about nursing autonomy, some of these advocates rely on the views of workplace sociologists rather than nursing leaders and scholars. But there is a difference between having less power and being subordinate, which suggests that one party reports to another in a formal sense, i.e., a master-servant relationship. Physicians are no more the conceptual "masters" of nurses than the United States is the master of India. Just as human rights do not cease to exist simply because they are not fully observed, nursing autonomy does not cease to exist simply because it is subject to daunting practical constraints.

Career seekers who have the qualities nursing requires value autonomy greatly. It is not hard to see why they would have little interest in the mute, servile "nurses" they see on television. They must understand that nurses' autonomous practice has, despite the prevailing belief that it does not exist, saved countless lives. Nursing has been a kind of shadowy superhero, saying little and doing much: the Dark Knight Nurse. But that must change if the profession is to meet the health challenges ahead.

# MEDIA PORTRAYALS OF THE NURSE AS AUTONOMOUS PROFESSIONAL

The most influential entertainment media regularly presents nurses as lowly physician handmaidens who are peripheral to serious health care. But some news and even entertainment items do convey some sense that nurses operate with autonomy.

## Nursing Authority in Television and Film
### BITCHES AND AUTONOMOUS PROFESSIONALS

Very little entertainment television presents nurses as autonomous. *ER* has at times shown its nurse characters working with a degree of independence. Of course, the show has also been the most persuasive purveyor of the handmaiden image, suggesting in many ways, some subtle, that nurses are ultimately responsible to physicians. But it's worth examining a few of the show's indications of nursing autonomy.

Once again, the most obvious recent examples are the late 2005 episodes with nurse manager Eve Peyton, discussed in chapter 3. Peyton was the first real nurse manager the show portrayed in any depth since the 1990s. She managed the ED nursing staff with authority and resisted physician care plans when necessary, though her management style did cause other characters to see her as a "bitch." Peyton upset chief resident Archie Morris by holding a nursing staff meeting (imagine!), and she embarrassed him with her superior clinical knowledge when he tried to break it up. Later a chastised Morris told fellow physicians that he could not interfere because nurses are "autonomous professionals." Peyton promoted major nurse character Sam Taggart to assistant nurse manager (a role the show promptly forgot about). Together, Peyton and Taggart abruptly fired veteran nurse Haleh Adams for working excessive overtime. Adams was later rehired, but the plotline suggested that hiring nurse managers and firing veteran nurses were fairly casual affairs. Peyton's departure in December 2005 was deeply flawed, as we will see in chapter 8, though she was at least fired by the "nursing supervisor."

Other *ER* episodes have also included indications of nursing autonomy. Examples include episodes in late 2006 and early 2007 with temporary nurse character Ben Parker. In one December 2006 episode, Taggart and Parker took the lead in caring for a homeless patient found on the street in the freezing Chicago winter. The interaction of two nurses with a patient is itself an extreme rarity: Hollywood nurses rarely speak to anyone but physicians. Taggart aggressively advocated for the patient, dressing down a manager from another hospital that had dumped the patient on the street and forcing that hospital to deliver the grateful patient to her parents' house an hour away. A November 2004 episode also had Taggart acting with autonomy in caring and advocating for a seriously injured rape victim, whose head and neck swelling prevented her from speaking clearly. Taggart was something like a full partner with her physician boyfriend Luka Kovac in caring for this patient. Taggart also displayed initiative in enabling the patient to give a police detective a description of her attacker, a procedure in which Taggart took the patient off the ventilator for short periods and deflated the tracheostomy balloon.

Another show that displayed significant nursing autonomy was the six-episode miniseries *RAN: Remote Area Nurse*, which aired on Australia's SBS-TV in early 2006. The drama's public health nurse Helen Tremaine was the only licensed health professional living on a Torres Strait island, and she provided a range of care on her own. Tremaine pushed back against a visiting physician's attempts to tell her what to do with an at-risk pregnant patient — "Since when does a registered nurse outrank a qualified physician?" — though there remained a sense that he was the ultimate health authority.

Some television documentaries have effectively conveyed nursing autonomy. The Discovery Health Channel documentaries *Lifeline: The Nursing Diaries* (2004) and *Nurses* (2002), discussed in chapter 3, showed skilled nurses working autonomously at major U.S. hospitals, suggesting that physicians do not direct nursing care. In addition, a 2003 episode of the National Geographic Channel's *Doctors Without Borders: Life in the Field*, a cable television series about the Nobel Prize-winning non-governmental organization, focused primarily on the work of its nurses. The episode included the stories of a veteran nurse running a health care system in an Ivory Coast prison, as well as nurses fighting tuberculosis during a refugee crisis in Sierra Leone and in a depressed region of Uzbekistan. One irony is that the name Doctors Without Borders sends a misleading message about the work of the organization: nurses are the most numerous health professionals among the group's workers.

## CONFRONTING THE ZOMBIES

A few recent films have conveyed a sense of nursing autonomy. Mike Nichols's *Angels in America* (2003) and Zack Snyder's *Dawn of the Dead* (2004), both discussed in chapter 3, featured strong major nurse characters providing vital health care with little or no physician involvement. In the apocalyptic zombie film, the nurse character Ana literally patches up and cares for her band of survivors with no skilled help at all. In Nichols's HBO adaptation of Tony Kushner's play, nurse Belize appears to be the only real health practitioner on his AIDS ward. When physician Henry comes to have his patient Roy Cohn admitted one night, Henry is annoyed that Belize does not jump to attention. Henry sniffs that nurses are supposed to wear white. Belize responds that physicians are supposed to be home in Westchester, asleep.

Nichols explored some similar territory in his 2001 HBO adaptation of Margaret Edson's play *Wit*. The film explores the tough but emotionally homeless scholar Vivian Bearing's confrontation with a life-threatening illness. The self-indulgent research physicians in *Wit* display blatant disregard for her well-being. Nurse Susie Monahan is not an intellectual, but she does want to provide Vivian with professional health care. This brings her into conflict with the physicians pushing Vivian's chemotherapy and heroic measures to prolong her life. Despite their differences, the two women form an important bond. Audra McDonald's performance as Susie is arguably a bit too meek, but she conveys a fiery core when she must stop the physicians from going against Bearing's wishes. (McDonald has moved on to play a heroic physician on *Private Practice*.)

Another area in which Hollywood has conveyed something of nursing autonomy is in recent films about World War II. Joe Wright's 2007 film adaptation of the 2003 novel *Atonement* follows Ian McEwan's characters into the carnage of World War II, and in doing so includes a look at British wartime nursing. The movie adds visuals to the book's powerful account of hospital care, showing the formidable authority of the senior nurses and the courage required of all the nurses caring for the horrifically wounded soldiers. Neither the film nor the book conveys much of the expertise that nursing requires, but both present nurse-centered visions of care in which physicians play virtually no role.

## True Colors in the News Media

Some of the lengthy press accounts of critical care nursing discussed in chapter 3 are also effective portrayals of nursing autonomy. John Blanton's April 2007 *Wall Street Journal* piece describing his experience as a new burn unit nurse gave readers a detailed account of nursing, with the physician role reduced to little more than a reference to the need to "keep a close eye on what doctors ordered" because "they make mistakes, too." Chris Colin's July 2007 *San Francisco Chronicle* piece about NICU nurses at the University of California at San Francisco likewise presented a critical care universe in which physicians did not really appear. And Scott Allen's October 2005 *Boston Globe* report about the intense ICU training of a new nurse similarly placed nurses at the core of patient care, though elements of that report did suggest that physicians were ultimately in charge. The value of these accounts is not that they suggest physicians' work does not matter, but that they show that nursing care is based on nurses' own unique scope of practice.

Two December 2004 items present nurses as the driving force in outpatient clinics. South Africa's *Star* ran a piece by Kerry Cullinan about the challenges faced by nurse managers at the legendary Alexandra Clinic, which handles chronic illnesses and labor and delivery in an overcrowded township. A column by Phillippa Stevenson in the *New Zealand Herald* paid tribute to palliative care nurse Cynthia Ward, founder and manager of True Colours, a new health service that "aims to support families at and from the moment their child is diagnosed with a chronic, serious or life-threatening illness."

Some reporting has examined nurse-physician power relations, with mixed results. In May 2006 a *HealthDay News* piece by Karen Pallarito described a new Johns Hopkins study suggesting that surgeons' teamwork is poor. Pallarito noted that ORs have historically been governed by a "pecking order" headed by the surgeon, who is seen as the "captain" of the ship, and that this hierarchy may discourage nurses from speaking up. Ironically, even though one study researcher was Hopkins's director of surgical nursing, the piece failed to include a single comment from a nurse, though it did discuss measures to ensure that nurses have the practical authority to increase patient safety.

In August 2005 Columbia physician Barron H. Lerner published an essay in the *New York Times*, "Practicing Medicine Without a Swagger," which had the unusual defect of *understating* physician power. It suggested that the days when physicians arrogantly "ruled the roost" "may have been fun" — no, really, that's what he wrote — but that today physicians are more likely to be treated as "employees" than "royalty." In the writer's view all that's left today are "periodic perks," like being addressed as "Doctor" and jumping to the front of lines for flu shots. Lerner deserves credit for discussing past abuses, but his piece offers a subtle whitewash of disruptive physician conduct, which threatens patient care. His post-royalty vision suggests that nurses are on the verge of enjoying practical authority commensurate with their conceptual autonomy. Maybe all they have to do is make "Barron" wait for his flu shot like everyone else.

Many press pieces showcase the autonomous work of public health nurses, including the articles about school nurses discussed in chapter 3. In addition, in July 2007 the *Copenhagen Post* ran an item about a "mobile nurse task force" — that is, two nurses on bicycles — who diagnose and treat most of their elderly patients' problems at the patients' homes, avoiding traumatic and costly hospital visits. January 2006 articles in New York newspapers discussed the shortage of Suffolk County public health nurses. A *Newsday* piece by Ridgely Ochs and a *New York Times* report by Julia C. Mead explained how the nurses improve patient outcomes, including reducing infant mortality rates. In January 2004 the *Toronto Star* ran Scott Simie's piece about the work of "street nurse" Cathy Crowe, one of Canada's most prominent advocates for the homeless.

Though Hollywood's depictions of military nurses have focused on the past, the news media has offered more current accounts of military nurses playing leadership roles. An October 2007 issue of *Time* magazine included a profile of U.S. Navy Commander Maureen Pennington, the "first nurse to lead a surgical company during combat operations." Caroline Kennedy's piece does not directly discuss Pennington's nursing skills, and it includes maternal imagery, but it also highlights her leadership. The field hospitals she led in her 2006 tour in Iraq had an "unprecedented" 98 percent survival rate.

In March 2007 National Public Radio ran a *Leading Ladies* profile, "Clara Adams-Ender: Army Achiever." Cheryl Corley interviewed the retired general, who headed the Army Nurse Corps from 1987 to 1991. Gen. Adams-Ender discussed her career and other issues, including the recently reported problems at Walter Reed Medical Center, where she once ran the department of nursing. The profile had little to say about nursing, however. Gen. Adams-Ender reportedly established the first neonatal ICU in Germany, but NPR failed to mention it. Still, the piece did show that nurses can lead at the highest levels.

## "NURSE, HAND ME MY LAPTOP": MEDIA PORTRAYALS OF THE NURSE AS HANDMAIDEN

In November 2007 Seattle's Group Health ran Internet ads for its "Ask the Doc" service, in which patients communicate with advanced practitioners by email. The tag line: "Nurse, hand me my laptop." Yes, maybe laptops are the new stethoscopes. But get your own laptop, buddy, we're busy saving lives. Of course, nurses do hand physicians things when care requires. However, these ads suggested that nurses are gofers whose use of advanced care technology consists mainly of handing it to physicians, the *real* health experts. But in hospital settings and many others, nurses are the main patient educators. Nurses at Group Health itself regularly communicate with patients by email!

Nurses at Group Health persuaded the company to pull the ad. But the popular media sends these same handmaiden messages every day. Influential entertainment television shows often portray authoritative physicians telling submissive nurses what to do. And especially since the great majority of nursing is rarely shown, these scenarios reinforce the prevailing notion that nursing is all about doing physicians' bidding.

## *ER:* "I'm the Doctor. This Is My Call."

*ER* is probably the most powerful modern source of the handmaiden image. That's because the series' hundreds of episodes have been shown around the world for so long, because its relatively realistic portrayal of hospital care is so persuasive, and because the skilled handmaiden image is so central to the show's nursing portrayal.

November 2007 *ER* episodes suggested that nurses report to physicians. One has chief of ED medicine Kevin Moretti implementing new triage policies and actually telling Taggart, "Sam, you're supposed to be covering triage right now." Taggart complies. In another scene, resident Tony Gates and Taggart lead some nurses through the ED explaining new policies, including treating pain at triage, and recording the Wong-Baker pain score. Gates: "Put it in your charts, the docs will be checking." Taggart is involved with this, but Gates is plainly the leader. These scenes tell viewers that physicians direct nurses and that physicians direct triage. In fact, nurse managers do that. And it is nurses who have led the way in pain management, despite decades of physician resistance.

Another plotline in the November 2007 episodes is about a precocious thirteen-year-old named Josh, who is dying of an incurable neurological disorder. The boy wants to avoid the ventilator, and Gates clears that idea with his attending and the hospital's ethics office — but not the boy's mother or Taggart. When Taggart sees this plan presented to the boy's mother as a foregone conclusion, she objects. Outside, Gates informs the veteran nurse how nasty vents are, no doubt based on his superior knowledge of ventilator care and his more holistic approach. (We're kidding.) Gates contemptuously tells Taggart that they will not be intubating. Taggart starts to call the ethics line, but Gates says he's already discussed it with ethics, then grabs the phone from Taggart and slams it down, yelling, "Stop! I'm the doctor. This is my call. Now you can either mix this morphine drip or you can take yourself off this case, because we're done here." Taggart stalks off. As is usually the case when *ER* physicians dismiss nurses like this, Taggart has no answer, leaving the impression that although Gates was harsh, what he says is correct — major care decisions are indeed "his call." The story shows Taggart as a spirited patient advocate and educator, but also as a somewhat myopic subordinate who can be excluded from key care discussions, and who must ultimately give way to the holistic, end-of-life wisdom of the *physicians*. This incident also functions as a turning point in Gates's development. Uppity nurse Sam thinks she can tell Dr. Gates what to do because he's just a resident, but our little resident is growing fast, learning to be a *real* physician.

Even the late 2005 Eve Peyton episodes included handmaiden messages. The October episodes indicated that Peyton did not report to the chief of ED medicine but that she and the other ED nurses reported to the hospital's overall chief of medicine Kerry Weaver. In the scene in which chief resident Morris wanted to stop Peyton from having a nurse staff meeting, Weaver let him know that only she had the power to stop it. But Weaver was never identified as the chief executive officer, and so she would have no authority over nurse managers like Peyton. In addition, the December 2005 episode in which Peyton got fired began with new chief of ED medicine Luka Kovac sending three ED nurses home — and calling them "support staff" — because he foresaw a light shift.

Other examples of handmaiden imagery, sometimes subtle, stretch back into the show's extraordinarily long history. A September 2005 episode acknowledged that veteran nurses play a role in coping with "July syndrome," which occurs when new physicians arrive in U.S. hospitals to begin their internships. Nurse character Chunie Marquez prevented several dangerous intern errors, and Haleh Adams critiqued a new second-year resident's intern teaching. But rather than teaching the junior physicians, as real nurses often do, the veteran nurse characters simply reported the problems to the senior physicians, as if their responsibility was to the senior physicians, not patients.

A February 2004 episode showed Taggart's autonomous care for a young sexual abuse victim, but it also presented then-chief of ED medicine Weaver as Taggart's functional manager. In the episode, the patient's fiancé and his friends have impregnated her in an abusive encounter that seems a lot like gang rape. When Taggart confronts the fiancé, he grabs her and refuses to let go. She decks him with some serious martial arts skills. The man appears to have no serious injuries, but the show regards it as excessive force. Weaver tells Taggart that a visiting human resources consultant has recommended that she be fired. Weaver also says she knows Taggart had similar problems at past jobs. Weaver says the "director of nursing" will speak with Taggart, but the rest of the scene conveys that Weaver is in charge. No actual nurse manager appears, because on the show, physicians are the real nurse managers.

The show made that situation clear in an astonishing October 2003 episode. In that one, many veteran ED nurses stage a walkout when they learn that the hospital plans to cut them back to part time and hire supposedly cheaper travelers and new graduates who will work for "minimum wage" (don't ask). As a result of the walkout, chief of ED medicine Robert Romano summarily fires six nurses. Then-nurse Lockhart tells Romano that he "can't fire nurses." Romano says he can if they walk off the job. To this Lockhart has no real response. There is no evident involvement from any nursing manager. In another scene, ER physician Susan Lewis forbids Lockhart to tell a teenage girl that she has a fatal heart/lung condition, at the behest of the girl's parents. The girl is panicked because she is getting clues that something serious is wrong with her, but no one will tell her the truth. Lewis impatiently reminds Lockhart that Lewis is the patient's physician, Lockhart is the patient's nurse, and so Lockhart must do what Lewis says. Lockhart has — you guessed it — no response except to look hurt. Lewis is harsh but apparently correct.

## Grey's Anatomy:
## "You Know Why I Stopped Being a Nurse?"

No one could possibly think, from watching Grey's Anatomy, that nurses were anything but physician subordinates. Nurse characters have, very rarely, questioned physician care plans. But the vast majority of nurses who appear are silent, submissive servants. Time and again, the show has told viewers that the nurses report to physicians. Nurses on Grey's do display resentment and petty vindictiveness when they are abused by their physician masters. But that is not the same as being an autonomous professional.

In a May 2008 episode, Seattle Grace's nurses boycott all surgeries of plastic surgeon Mark "McSteamy" Sloane because he has loved and left too many of them. The nurses actually complain to their union, and a union rep shows up to get chief of surgery Richard Webber to force all physicians and nurses to submit the names of their sexual contacts. Among other things, this is a clear suggestion that the chief of surgery manages nurses. Finally, chief resident Miranda Bailey calls about forty of the nurses together in the hospital atrium to publicly chastise them and get them back to work. Bailey disparages McSteamy as a "whore" but allows that he's a good surgeon, and she stresses that the nurses all knew what his reputation was, so "let us all close our knees and get back to our jobs." Not a single nurse can reply. Bailey shouts "Disperse!" and the nurse-sheep amble back to their pastures.

The January 2007 episode in which Sloane praises nurses also has him punishing the interns by dumping nurses' apparently disgusting work — debriding bedsores — on the interns. Presumably, he directs both interns and nurses. Sloane's statement that the nurses are "helpful" actually reinforces damaging assumptions. Of course "helpful" is a good thing in general, but this comment in context suggests that nurses are helpful in the physician mission of providing all meaningful health care, rather than in providing autonomous nursing care. And "helpful" is pretty faint praise for life-saving health professionals. Would anyone suggest that physicians, as a class, are "helpful"?

In a September 2006 episode, nurse Tyler smugly informs intern Cristina that he was part of a team that just saved a life in a code. But Tyler tells Cristina only to justify his failure to earn the $20 she paid him to act as a lookout so she could have sex with her boyfriend, a surgeon, in his hospital bed. Tyler seems to get the last laugh, but he's still a lackey who accepts $20 tips for tasks other than his real job. Later, Tyler pages intern George O'Malley to tell him that a cancer patient has been shoplifting and is planning to leave without having her operation. Then Tyler steps back to let George handle the important psychosocial issues. Plainly, Tyler works for George, not the patient.

The January 2006 nurse's strike episodes repeatedly tell viewers that the nurses report to the chief of surgery. These episodes make a few points about short-staffing and forced overtime. But the episodes present the nurses as bitter serfs, and suggest that nursing is mostly about paperwork, room assignments, and trivial patient quirks. And the episodes make a joke out of O'Malley's sympathy for the nurses. The chief of surgery's "assistant" Patricia is described as someone who "used to" be a nurse; as noted in chapter 3, nursing is not seen as a profession but merely something physical you do at the bedside. But now, as assistant to the chief, Patricia manages the nursing crisis. After all, the show has no nurse managers. Patricia stops to lecture the temporary nurses about how the patient charts are organized by room number, then addresses nearby attending surgeons Burke and Shepherd: "You know why I stopped being a nurse? Doctors. Doctors who don't know how to pitch in." These two surgeons tell the chief he should resolve the strike, but the chief says it would take $2 million per year to hire the extra nurses needed to address the overtime issue. Finally, the chief admits to Patricia that "we" need the nurses. She suggests they forgo a surgical robot the chief recently ordered, and he reluctantly agrees. The chief appears outside the hospital shaking hands with the nurses and congratulating them.

And an April 2005 episode presented scrub nurses as the loyal appendages of surgeons. The nurse, a dying pancreatic cancer patient named Elizabeth Fallon, was formidable and savvy. She had worked for decades with Ellis Grey, the legendary surgeon mother of lead character Meredith. Ellis recalled that Fallon was an "excellent" nurse, whatever that means. But Fallon was also seen as a career physician appendage, focused on gruffly charting the progress of the physicians around her, like a drill sergeant training bright young things like Cristina to be officers. Fallon's remark that she was "Ellis's scrub nurse for eighteen years" is a slap in the face to peri-operative nurses, who are professionals with their own science-based scope of practice. Nurses work with surgeons, not for them.

## *House*: Help! Golems Are Loose in the Hospital!

Nurse characters on *House* probably speak and do even less than nurses on the other major Hollywood hospital shows, and as a result, the show's handmaiden portrayal may be the most absolute. The vast majority of nurse appearances involve a character popping up out of nowhere to absorb a physician command, like the golems of Jewish folklore — mute, brainless humanoids crafted from inanimate material for basic tasks by the wisest and holiest, notably early rabbis. Recall from chapter 3 that House himself joked during a "playing God" monologue in a November 2005 episode that cleanup tasks were why he had "created nurses." From time to time the show also shows a nurse acting as a silent administrative assistant to "dean of medicine" Lisa Cuddy.

In the April 2008 episode with the nurses' strike plotline, House glibly says he does not "use nurses." House could have said he doesn't "practice" with nurses, or (translating into House-speak) that he wouldn't let those fools with Daffy Duck on their clothes get near his patients. But "use" suggests that nurses are just physician tools. The show confirms this attitude in an exchange between House and Cuddy in which both physicians indicate that Cuddy is in charge of the striking nurses. In fact, dealing with the nurses would presumably be the job of the CEO and the chief nursing officer. But *House* has no nurse managers.

A May 2007 episode also underlined the nurses' handmaiden role on the show. The complete dialogue of the nurse characters in this episode is as follows: "Yes, doctor." "Right away." "I was just trying to get a urine sample, and he went crazy!" These lines reflect a vision of handmaidens who perform menial tasks but panic in an emergency, relying on physicians to supply all thinking, expertise, and courage. At one point House enters Cuddy's office. She sits at her desk with some paperwork, as a nurse in scrubs stands beside her. House: "You girls can gossip later." A moment later, when the nurse has not left, House addresses her: "When I said you girls can gossip later, I was throwing you out in a polite way." Cuddy hands some paperwork to the nurse and makes a face suggesting, "You know how he is, we'll come back to this later." The nurse leaves without a word. After Cuddy and House banter a while, Cuddy sends House away: "Send in Nurse Unger on your way out." Yes, House trashes everyone, but the difference is that we can see that physicians like Cuddy are smart and able, and they deal it back to House in spades. The nurses slink away like wounded mice.

In a February 2007 episode, physician Cameron is providing solo bedside care to a patient with the rare condition CIPA (congenital insensitivity to pain with anhidrosis). The patient starts seizing. Cameron presses a button, saying "Call a code," then seems to note the patient's high temperature. She yells, "Need ice packs and cooling blankets!" A nurse arrives, and Cameron says, "Got saline in there?" The nurse actually starts to argue: "She's not flushed, she's not sweaty, you must be —" Cameron cuts her off: "She has a temperature of 105." That silly nurse needs to listen to the physicians who provide bedside care! This is a rare *House* scene in which a nurse actually questions a physician command, but she's not helpful. Nurses on the show are sniping ninnies who don't see the big picture, or they're bureaucrats who are afraid to take responsibility and must await physician authority.

A May 2006 episode offers excellent examples of the show's "golem" portrayal, with nurses effectively conjured into existence to perform unskilled tasks. At one point physician Chase is with a patient and her father. Giving the patient a chelating agent by

IV to help her body dispose of unwanted iron, Chase explains the procedure to the father. The nurse who would actually perform and explain this task is not there. The patient goes into respiratory distress, and a monitor beeps. Chase calmly says, "Crash cart." Within five seconds, two nurses are in the room with a crash cart. One of the nurses hands Chase an intubation tool and he saves the patient's life. Throughout, the nurses say nothing. Later House is alone with this patient and her father. No one else is shown in the room. The intubated patient suddenly has a breathing problem. House wants to eject the father, ostensibly so he can do some scary procedure (actually he just wants to continue berating the patient). House turns to a nurse, who simply was not there before, and commands, "Get him out of here." The nurse mutely complies. After all, she serves House, and there is but one House.

## Shut Up and Follow Orders: Nursing on Other Health Care Shows

Other health care shows have done no better than the major ones in portraying nursing autonomy, and in some cases they have been worse.

The early episodes of *Private Practice*, in late 2007, presented nurse Dell as a receptionist at an LA clinic. Dell was plainly an assistant to the clinic physicians, with no scope of practice and no unique expertise to add to the show's "heroic physician" narrative. Because Dell was studying to be a midwife, he was eager to learn what the main character, star ob-gyn Addison Montgomery, could teach him. The September 2007 series premiere included scenes in which Dell, helping Montgomery with a delivery, came off as an eager but ignorant layperson — as if he had never cared for a patient and needed Montgomery to tell him everything. Well, he did hold the patient's hand on his own initiative, and notice that she had passed out. Alert viewers could also catch glimpses of wallpaper nurses in the background of the episodes, but it was not clear if any of them would ever display the ability to speak, much less think.

*Scrubs* also generally presents its physician characters as directing nurses and nursing care. It has repeatedly told viewers that the nurses ultimately report to chief of medicine Bob Kelso, though it has also suggested that nurse Carla Espinosa, who provides direct care, is a "head nurse." As noted in chapter 3, in a February 2007 episode Kelso took over for Espinosa as a nurse manager while she was on maternity leave.

An extraordinary November 2003 *Scrubs* episode purported to teach Carla that nursing is all about shutting up and doing what physicians tell you. In the episode, Carla advised resident physician Elliot to give a patient a certain drug, which Elliot did. The patient developed a paradoxical reaction, and Elliot was furious. She told Carla that Carla should never have spoken up and that Elliott's job was to ignore Carla and do whatever Elliott thought was right. Carla's fiancé, surgical resident Turk, told Carla how a surgical nurse with twenty years experience had recently tried to tell him what kind of suture knot to tie. He said he had kicked the nurse out of the OR and made her cry, because in the hospital, physicians are in charge. Turk said the job of nurses is to follow physician "orders," because ultimately the physicians are responsible for the patients (and presumably nurses are not). Thus, Carla had no business giving Elliott advice. Carla accepted this judgment. The final scene of the story found Elliott and Carla at a patient's bedside. Elliot asked for a certain treatment. Carla meekly obeyed, smiling, clearly relieved to have learned her proper role as physician helpmate. There was no irony in this megalomaniacal fantasy, which was especially insidious because Carla endorsed it.

*Strong Medicine* included nurse midwife character Peter Riggs, who at times displayed limited autonomy. But even his intermittent appearances were undermined by a persistent vision of physicians as the masters of all health care. And other nurses — when they appeared at all — were almost always faceless servants, silent and submissive. Indeed, outside Peter's occasional plotlines, nursing was either not shown or was performed by the physicians. One January 2002 episode about a nursing strike actually did convey the deadly effects of nurse short-staffing, and made the point that physicians could not easily do nurses' jobs. But even this episode made clear that the physicians were in charge. As one striking nurse said (wrongly), physicians are management and nurses are labor. Riggs led the striking nurses, negotiating directly with a physician who appeared to be both chief of medicine and hospital CEO, but no nurse manager ever appeared.

## "I'll Go Get the Doctor!": Nursing on Non-Health Care Shows

As you might expect, some of the worst handmaiden portrayals of nursing appear in shows that are not mainly about health care. And it's not just cliché-ridden sitcoms.

An April 2008 episode of ABC's *Desperate Housewives* presented a nurse as a mousy physician lackey who could be bribed into revealing sensitive patient information with a free lunch. In the episode, character Gaby's boyfriend Carlos is an inpatient with an eye injury, which only Carlos knows will mean permanent blindness. Another of Carlos's girlfriends, the notorious Edie, visits him in the hospital. Edie gets angry when Carlos admits the diamonds in a bracelet he gave her are fake. Walking down the hall, Edie spots a nurse eating a sandwich. Edie asks when Carlos will get his sight back. Nurse: "I don't know…Mr. Solis's condition is very serious…" Edie: "Serious? What's wrong?" Nurse: "Well…you know, you should really talk to the doctor about this. I don't even think his girlfriend knows." The nurse suggests she has "said too much already," but then she succumbs to Edie's offer to treat her to lunch at a "great little French bistro." Edie easily gets information out of the unsophisticated nurse. Meanwhile, Gaby brings a priest to the hospital and marries Carlos, but Carlos hides the fact that his blindness is permanent. Edie later delights in informing Gaby, who is livid. The timid nurse is evidently there to act as a pass-through to the physicians. She can't speak with any real authority, even to say the law and her own ethics limit her ability to speak about the patient. Instead, she does the classic hand-maiden thing: pass the buck to the physician who has real power and expertise.

Late 2007 episodes of Larry David's HBO sitcom *Curb Your Enthusiasm* also presented nurses as handmaidens. In an October episode, "The N Word," a black surgeon overhears Larry relating a story in which another white man had used that racist word. The furious surgeon, wrongly assuming Larry is the bigot, takes revenge on the next white man in his path by shaving the head of his patient, who happens to be Larry's friend Jeff. In the OR, a nurse weakly tries to stop the surgeon but ends up obediently handing him the clippers after the surgeon orders her to do so. Another nurse tries to cover up what the surgeon did, suggesting to Jeff's wife that it was accidental, before the surgeon orders her from their room so he can apologize.

In a November 2007 episode, Larry is reluctant to tell a nurse at a gastroenterology office about a sensitive condition, arguing that he'll just have to tell the physician again (which he does). The nurse responds not by describing her skill and autonomy but by claiming unpersuasively that the system saves important physician time. It's not that these scenarios could not happen, but presenting only these visions of nursing reinforces handmaiden stereotypes.

A July 2005 episode of HBO's *Six Feet Under* suggested that nurses basically help the smart physicians who provide all important care. In the episode, character Nate Fisher is taken to an LA-area hospital after collapsing because of a brain hemorrhage. Nate has an operation to stop the bleeding, though he remains in a coma. Meanwhile, family and friends gather, including Brenda, his pregnant wife. The family deals with two physicians before Nate's operation, including a neurosurgeon who tells them what they can expect. The surgeon also appears afterward to answer questions, noting that it could be weeks before Nate emerges from his coma. Both physicians are polite, knowledgeable, and reasonably sensitive. The next morning, Nate is on a med-surg floor with only Brenda present. Nate suddenly wakes up. Brenda calls for the nearby nurse. The nurse sees Nate and responds, "I'll go get the doctor!" No smile, no support, no assessment, no patient interaction. The nurse flees the room. She is a terrified flunky.

## News Media Helpers

The entertainment media is the leading source of explicit handmaiden imagery, but echoes of it can be found in the news media, which often at least implies that physicians direct all hospital care. Indeed, the implication of the May 2007 *New York Times* piece about Gov. Jon Corzine's recovery from a car crash and many other press reports discussed in chapter 3 is that physicians manage nurses (and everyone else). Even some articles that highlight nursing skill, such as Scott Allen's October 2005 *Boston Globe* report about the ICU training of a new nurse, fall into this trap to some extent. Likewise, the February 2007 *New York Times* Crossword Puzzle clue "I.C.U.

helpers" suggested that nurses are physician assistants, rather than central players in intensive care.

Consider a story posted in September 2006 on the ABC News website about dangerously long emergency department waits. An Illinois woman was found dead in an ED waiting room two hours after a nurse told her to wait. The coroner found that the woman had shown "classic symptoms of a heart attack," and the coroner's jury ruled the death a homicide. The piece highlights the serious potential consequences of triage errors, and it also links the apparent problem in this case to ED overcrowding. But the report seems to wrongly assume that physicians are ultimately responsible for all ED care. It relies solely on comments from the American College of Emergency Physicians. And a statement attributed to the president of ACEP advises dissatisfied patients to talk to the triage nurse, but if that "doesn't work," to "ask to speak to the emergency physician." This advice gives the mistaken impression that ED nurses report to physicians. In fact, patients in such a situation should generally ask to speak with the charge nurse, the clinical nurse specialist, or the ED nurse manager. Nurses are the triage leaders.

# CHAPTER 5

# The Naughtiest Nurse

IN THE EARLY 1990S an inebriated homeless patient assaulted an emergency department nurse at a public hospital in San Francisco. The patient grabbed her breast. In the late 1990s exactly the same thing happened to that nurse while she was working at a major private hospital in Washington, DC — except that the assaulting patient was a United States ambassador to a foreign nation. The nurse was Sandy.

Contrary to the "naughty nurse" image, nurses do not wish to be sexualized, harassed, or assaulted. In a December 2005 study, University of Missouri communications professor Debbie Dougherty found that more than 70 percent of the nurses she surveyed in four states had been sexually harassed by patients.[1] In March 2006, Dougherty told a writer for the *Monster* website that she was "surprised" at the aggression the nurses faced: "Patients threatened to attack nurses sexually and called them prostitutes." A 2002 *NurseWeek* study found that 19 percent of nurses had been sexually harassed in the previous year.[2] Sexual abuse has a negative impact on patient care, as a December 2005 Associated Press item about Dougherty's study noted.[3] A nurse traumatized by abuse cannot provide her best care. And as nurses quoted in a June 2007 State House News Service (Boston) piece made clear, abused nurses often do not receive adequate support from their hospital employers. Some employers seem to view even life-threatening abuse as part of the nurses' job. Just get over it!

Much of global society continues to regard nurses as sex objects. An August 2006 Agence France Presse item reported that a recent poll had found that 54 percent of British men had sexual fantasies about nurses — more than about any other profession. Nursing led a list of traditionally female, service-oriented jobs; it was followed by maids and flight attendants. By contrast, the poll found that women's popular fantasies focused on traditionally male jobs associated with heroism and/or socioeconomic power, including medicine. Leading that list were "firemen," about whom 47 percent of British women dreamed. For men, it seems, to be the object of fantasies is a mark of power and prestige. For women, it is a mark of perceived submissiveness and low status.

The image of the naughty nurse is a common cultural reference. In March 2007, on *Live with Regis and Kelly*, Kelly Ripa repeatedly promised to be a "sponge bath nurse" in her "little nursey costume" for co-host Regis Philbin, who was undergoing bypass surgery. Ripa's comments were enthusiastically amplified in press stories about Philbin's condition, from the Associated Press to the *New York Post*.

After nurses persuaded shoe company Skechers to stop including images of pop star Christina Aguilera dressed as a naughty nurse in global ad campaigns in 2004, Aguilera posed for photos in a naughty nurse costume at her October 2005 Las Vegas Halloween party. As *People* reported and the photos confirmed, she was "playing doctor" with her scrubs-clad music executive fiancé. Take that, little nursies! And in December 2006, sometime Italian prime minister and media mogul Silvio Berlusconi found a novel way to thank his nurses at the Cleveland Clinic, where he had just had a pacemaker implanted: "Italian nurses are better-looking…. These ones scare me a bit. Don't even think about leaving me alone at night with one of them."

In August 2004 the *Times* of London reported that in "some Asian cultures, nursing is considered on a par with prostitution." In June 2006 the Inter Press Service News Agency quoted the press secretary of the Pakistan Nurses Association as noting that "the majority of patients and their relatives regard us as sex symbols." That story described sexual assaults by patients and physicians about which nothing was done. One nurse found that "not even paramedics" would marry her because, she explained, her hospital colleagues "think I am a prostitute."

The media plays a central role in perpetuating the global vision of nurses as half-dressed nymphomaniacs. From the time the modern naughty nurse image emerged in the 1960s, as discussed in chapter 2, the prevalence of the image has been staggering. It appears in television shows, pop music videos, sexually oriented products, and the news media. Major corporations have used the image to sell products such as beer, vodka, razor blades, cosmetics, shoes, men's underwear, milk, cell phone service, gum, vodka, and beer.

How sexualized is the media image of nurses? One easy way to measure is with the Internet.

### GOOGLE RESULTS FOR SELECTED
### ENGLISH LANGUAGE PHRASES — JUNE 2008

|  | "Sexy _____" | "Hot _____" | "Naughty _____" |
|---|---|---|---|
| "Lawyers" | 1,400 | 2,700 | 400 |
| "Doctors" | 13,400 | 8,400 | 3,600 |
| "Nurses" | 578,000 | 151,000 | 336,000 |

The naughty nurse image is not limited to straightforward indications that nurses are bimbos. It encompasses more subtle messages that nurses, who are primarily women, are mainly focused on the romantic pursuit of men, particularly physicians. Recall the May 2008 episode of *Grey's Anatomy* in which nurses actually boycotted the surgeries of surgeon Mark "McSteamy" Sloane because he had romanced then abandoned too many of them. The absurd plotline, discussed in chapter 4, suggested that nurses are losers grasping at any attractive physician.

Why are nurses so naughty? As explained in chapters 1 and 2, nurses have struggled since the founding of the modern profession to put society at ease with the idea of females providing intimate care to men. The profession's image has long teetered between extremes of femininity, from the angel to the harlot. It may be that some cannot get past the "madonna and whore" dichotomy: as females who provide intimate care, nurses must be one or the other. As the research suggests, and even a cursory look at the Internet confirms, male sexual fantasies often focus on traditionally female professions that are seen as involving basic personal services. These workers may be perceived as submissive females who are more sexually available or ripe for abuse because they have no strong, independent professional identity — not much else going for them. Some have also suggested that regarding nurses as sluts may help vulnerable male patients handle the fact that female nurses have some power over them. Illness and incapacity are frightening, and some may express that fear by diminishing the nearest available women.

Whatever the reasons, such social contempt discourages practicing and potential nurses, undermines nurses' claims to clinical and educational resources, and encourages workplace sexual abuse. The naughty nurse image is a factor in the nursing crisis, and overcoming it is key to resolving the shortage. Nurses have urged the media to reconsider its rampant use of the image. We just hope there's some other way to sell men beer and stuff.

## "PENNY SHOTS FOR NAUGHTY NURSES": WHY THE NAUGHTY NURSE MATTERS

In April 2008 a nursing student reported that a bar on Pittsburgh's South Side had been running the following promotion: "Penny Shots for Naughty Nurses."

The naughty nurse image might be good for some free drinks and social activities, but nurses and their patients pay in the long run. And one way they pay is in the loss of respect and resources nurses really need — pennies for nurses!

Naughty nurse images add to the chronic underfunding of nursing research, education, and clinical practice. Health care decision makers — many of whom are sadly uninformed about what nursing really is — are less likely to devote scarce resources to a profession that has become so degraded in the public mind. This negative image also holds little appeal for career seekers. The naughty nurse isn't just promiscuous. She's either submissive and dim, or else comically aggressive or evil. And she's always female. If a profession is constantly associated with female sexuality, it's not going to attract and retain many men. Nursing remains more than 90 percent female. When you combine the lack of respect, the low appeal to the more powerful gender, the intense training nursing actually requires, and the difficulty and stress of real nursing practice, it's no surprise that the profession remains in the midst of a global shortage. This is the difference between sexual images of female nurses and, say, female FBI agents, or for that matter, male firefighters. Those challenging professions are not being undermined by the idea that their members are sex-crazed twits. Nursing is.

Of course, there's nothing wrong with being seen as sexy — as long as that's not your dominant image in the workplace. An article published in *Psychology of Women Quarterly* in late 2005, based on research by Lawrence University professor Peter Glick, suggested that more sexualized work attire actually lessens respect for female workers in responsible jobs like management, causing others to see them as less competent and intelligent.[4] Constantly associating nursing with sex has the same effect.

Consider the inordinate amount of sexual abuse that nurses suffer at work. It's hard to prove the extent to which such abuse is caused by naughty nurse stereotyping, but it is reasonable to believe that the image has a real-world effect. If a profession is an object of endless sexual mockery and contempt, that status will invite sexual abuse, especially from those who are mentally altered, such as by drugs or mental illness.

Some say that naughty nurse imagery is just a "joke" or "fantasy" and no one believes nurses really are that way. Of course most people probably don't think the average nurse goes to work in lingerie, looking for sex. And it may be hard to see how one naughty nurse image could matter. But each image is a tiny part of a global wave of media imagery, all suggesting nursing is about hot females bestowing sexual favors. In the aggregate, decades of that message will have an impact. Even humor and fantasy images affect how people act, as explained in chapter 2. And suggesting that nurses are primarily sex objects in turn conveys the idea that nursing work consists of satisfying the sexual needs of patients and/or physicians, or at best, that nursing is so unimportant that nurses have time to focus on sex while caring for patients. Few people would accept "just joking" as an excuse for stereotyping of other disempowered groups.

Some claim that objections to the constant association of nursing with sex indicate prudishness. But there is a big difference between objecting to sexual images generally and objecting to the use of nursing as a marker for shallow, servile, sexually available females. The naughty nurse targets a life-saving profession in crisis.

Of course, sexual desires and fantasies do not instantly go away just because certain media images become less prevalent. But we doubt that something as specific in time as the naughty nurse image of recent decades is biologically predetermined or unchangeable, at least on a society-wide basis. It seems to us that the image is largely the result of specific cultural information, though it may incorporate some broader elements, such as the eroticism of apparent innocence. Some aspects of human attraction may evolve over time. For instance, common standards of human beauty do not appear to be the same today as in past centuries. It is in humanity's long-term interest to consider new ways to think about nurses.

One could argue that the work of nurses is so intimate that it will always be subject to some level of sexual fantasy. But the work of physicians is intimate, and they don't seem to suffer from the idea that they are submissive and sexually available.

At ground level, the devaluation of nursing translates into an underpowered profession that may not be strong enough to save your life when you need it to do so. The naughty nurse isn't going to catch deadly medication errors, intervene when a patient is about to crash, or teach a patient how to survive with a life-threatening condition. It's time for her to change into something a little more comfortable.

# CALL ME MAGDALENE: IS NURSING THE WORLD'S OLDEST PROFESSION?

Naughty nurse images circle the globe. As the rest of this chapter shows, virtually all are just variations on the tired bimbo imagery that has permeated pop culture since the 1960s. However, recently there have been fairly thoughtful media explorations of the naughty nurse image. Well, actually, we can think of just two examples. But hey — there are two!

One is Richard Prince's "nurse paintings," which were the subject of prominent exhibitions throughout the 2000s. Prince starts with the covers of mid-twentieth-century pulp novels that show the standing figure of a white-uniformed nurse. Then he covers much of the nurses' faces with white mask-like paint blobs. In many cases, red paint bleeds off different parts of the figures. Parts of the original book cover backgrounds emerge in vague, often ominous forms. Thus we get *Nympho Nurse*, *Aloha Nurse*, *Tender Nurse*, and the especially gory *Man Crazy Nurse #2* — which sold at Christie's New York for $7.4 million in May 2008. Many nurses object to Prince's paintings, and the artist could be accused of using misogynist iconography to score cheap pop art shock points. But it is hard to miss the irony driving the works. Prince's nurses are effectively gagged; they are literally defined by the large, aggressively ridiculous book titles, and they are alone in a world of scary shadows and blood. Trapped in their oppressive clothes and our oppressive attitudes, the pulp nurses may reflect the plight of today's real nurses, and of women generally. The blood spots on their bodies are stigmata of caring. The masks in particular point to critical problems today's nurses face, namely their invisibility and difficulty in speaking up for themselves. In some of the paintings, the nurses' eyes burn out over the mask, suggesting sentient beings struggling to assert a genuine identity.

A related example is the alternative band Sonic Youth's 2004 album *Sonic Nurse*, which used Prince's nursing imagery to explore troubling aspects of women's lives. The CD package art has images of the nurse paintings. Maybe the band saw nursing as a busy intersection on the boulevard of broken female dreams. The album title may also suggest that the band is not unlike a nurse, assessing a given environment and, in some sense, intervening. The song "Dude Ranch Nurse" is based on a Prince painting that in turn seems to be drawn from a 1953 Cherry Ames novel, one in a series of nursing adventures aimed at schoolgirls. The band's Kim Gordon sings that the "dude ranch dream has fallen apart," but still, "I could love him."

Unfortunately, the vast majority of naughty nurse imagery won't be telling the public anything useful about nursing. Consider some examples from recent advertising, television and film, sexually oriented media, pop music, and news media.

## Catching "Lusty-Nurse Fever": The Nurse in Global Advertising

The naughty nurse is especially adept at selling products to young men. But it seems she can sell anything, including women's shoes. She has even volunteered to promote non-profit endeavors.

The naughty nurse is eager for men to buy alcohol, even though real nurses spend much of their time handling the damage caused by alcohol abuse. Maybe it's all about nursing job security! First, of course, there's beer. In 2002 Colorado brewer Coors ran a Zima (colorless beer) television commercial depicting a "dream date" in which a female "nurse" in a revealing uniform played submissive temptress to a young male "physician." During the mid-2000s, Coors's Canadian division relied heavily on naughty nurse imagery in its Coors Light Trauma Tour, a marketing campaign based on sponsorship of extreme sports events. Naughty nurse models not only appeared in visual ads but also interacted with spectators at the events.

The naughty nurse also wants us to enjoy vodka irresponsibly. In 2006 Constellation Brands marketed its Hydra Vodka Water beverage with a Water Made Naughty campaign featuring a print ad with a naughty nurse underwater in a very short dress. Naughty nurse models also appeared at events promoting the drink.

Meanwhile, the maker of Gzhelka vodka (which appears to be the Russian government) crafted our favorite naughty nurse ad *ever*. In the television spot, which apparently started airing in 2006, an attractive young female nurse enters a hospital room. We hear the ominous theme from the 1968 thriller *Twisted Nerve*. The evil character Elle Driver whistled that theme in Quentin Tarantino's *Kill Bill* (2003); disguised as a nurse, she prepared to assassinate the hospitalized Bride character by lethal injection. But the Gzhelka nurse has something else in mind. She gives an IV bolus of a bottle of vodka to her unconscious male patient. Once the vodka starts infusing, the patient becomes very aroused under the sheet. The nurse mounts and has energetic intercourse with the still-unconscious patient. Onscreen text says there is "no prescription needed," and the nurse asks why the [obscenity] anyone would need medicine at all. Note the cool public health themes of a nurse/prostitute pushing huge quantities of vodka as a sexual aid and overall health promoter.

The naughty nurse has sold young males more health-oriented drinks as well. In 2008 Canada's Neilson Dairy marketed its Ultimate flavored milk products with a campaign that was remarkably similar to the earlier Coors Light Trauma Tour. Naughty nurse models appeared in ads and at an extreme sports tour. Neilson ads matched the "nurses" — the "Ultimate Recovery Team" — with sports-related sexual innuendo. In August 2008 the Registered Nurses Association of Ontario helped the company recover from its naughty nurse work-out, persuading it to remove the nurse element from the campaign.

The naughty nurse also wants her man to be well-groomed and sweetly scented before she provides her, you know, "nursing services." In late 2006 a print ad campaign for Schick's Quattro Titanium razor featured an injured male skateboarder in a research facility bed. He was surrounded by white-coated researchers — and three naughty "nurses" giving him "more intensive care." Schick placed the ad in *Sports Illustrated* and also distributed it at college bookstores, perhaps as an inspiration to nursing students. In a late 2005 television spot, Gillette's TAG Body Spray caused a provocatively dressed "nurse" to develop "highly contagious lusty-nurse fever" and climb into bed with a male patient wearing the product. In October 2007 Reuters reported that Unilever had angered a large nurses union by running billboard ads for Axe deodorant in major Spanish cities that showed a young "nurse" wearing a "short medical coat and stethoscope." And in September 2007 Cadbury Schweppes Canada ran television ads for Dentyne Ice chewing gum that showed female nurses being lured into bed with male patients the instant the men popped the product into their mouths. The tag line: "Get Fresh."

The naughty nurse also wants to show you a good time at bars and restaurants, often as part of an ironic health-related theme. In 2004 Los Angeles's Club Good Hurt began attracting patrons with local bands and "nurse" bartenders. The club's website advised poten-tial customers to "let our sexy nurses write your prescription for one of our signature drinks, like the Transfusion, and find out the true meaning of a Good Hurt."

In 2005 a Phoenix-area restaurant called the Heart Attack Grill began using scantily dressed naughty nurse waitstaff. The restaurant's marketing involved flaunting its anti-health menu, which included "quadruple-bypass" burgers and "flatliner fries." The "nurses" did "role playing": helping diners with "heart attacks," sitting on their laps, pushing the overfed in wheelchairs. However, Grill owner "Dr. Jon" Basso's "role" was to remain fully dressed, in a lab coat and tie. The Center for Nursing Advocacy thought the Grill was a striking example of the naughty nurse image, so in October 2006 it generated global press coverage about the restaurant.

The 2004 Skechers campaign, which was called "Naughty and Nice," featured Christina Aguilera wearing Skechers footwear in three different ads, including one in which she appeared both as a dominatrix naughty nurse and as the nurse's patient. Nurse Christina was about to inject patient Christina with a huge metal syringe connected to a big needle. This campaign ran in youth magazines and point-of-sale retail displays around the world, though nurses persuaded the company to drop the nurse ads.

And in July 2005 Reuters reported that the Spanish cosmetic surgery firm Corporación Dermoestética had used "50 mini-skirted models" dressed as nurses at its stock market share launch. It was unclear whether the models would also be caring for the firm's patients.

But the naughty nurse would be hurt if you thought she was all about money. Behind that sexy bra beats a passionate heart of caring! Just before the Halloween 2006 release of the horror film series installment *Saw III*, Lion's Gate and Twisted Pictures promoted a related blood drive with eye-catching posters featuring sexy/scary naughty nurse imagery. The film companies boasted of the lives their previous drives had saved, but these nurse images degraded the very professionals who use the blood collected to save those lives.

## "Cute Little Nurses": Modern Hollywood's Tribute

Although the state-of-the-art television image of nurses is the unskilled handmaiden, the naughty nurse certainly hasn't gone away. On the contrary, she has been a plot device on some of the most widely seen recent shows. In an October 2007 episode of *Desperate Housewives*, the sexy character Gaby donned naughty nurse attire as a cover to rub lotion on her husband, to covertly heal a case of the crabs she had given him. The naughty nurse also haunts recent horror films, helping to provide the required mix of fear, violence, and female sexuality.

The most notable prime-time television examples of naughty nurse imagery are on *Grey's Anatomy*. On *Grey's*, nurse characters have often been vehicles through which the show's pretty female physicians confront latent fears about female subservience and sexual virtue. December 2005 episodes displayed the fury of intern Izzie because the object of her affection, intern Alex, had call-room sex with less attractive nurse Olivia. Alex wants to talk, but Izzie snaps that he's "too busy screwing nurses to talk, just get out." At another point, intern Cristina marvels that "hell hath no fury like a girl whose non-boyfriend screws a nurse." Izzie also accuses Alex of having cheated on her with the "skanky syph nurse," a reference to the fact that Alex previously gave Olivia syphilis, which Olivia later passed on to intern George. Olivia had not known about the Alex and Izzie romance, and she is meekly apologetic to Izzie. In response, Izzie projects seething contempt.

These episodes reveal the interns' fears of sexual degradation and even of a kind of class miscegenation. Alex has not just cheated on Izzie, he has "screwed" a *nurse*, the low-rent embodiment of everything a smart, ambitious modern woman must avoid. Let's face it:

some people just don't belong. And we need not worry about being fair to them. Izzie calls Olivia a "skanky syph nurse" even though it was actually Alex who gave *Olivia* syphilis. And although Olivia slept with two interns, intern Meredith has apparently been getting drunk and sleeping with a different guy every night. Izzie does briefly call attention to this, but no one uses the expression "skanky syph doc." Worst of all, Alex's dalliance with Olivia indirectly associates Izzie herself with nursing.

*Grey's* has also found more comic uses for the naughty nurse. An October 2005 episode suggested that naughty nurse video pornography was a viable pain management tool, crediting a male patient's reliance on it. In the episode, Cristina actually expressed the view that such porn is misogynous, but evidently some women are more equal than others. When a storm knocked out the hospital's television system, she still created a verbal naughty nurse scenario for the patient, albeit reluctantly.

More recently, the show has relied more on the nurse-grasping-for-physician-love theme, as in the 2008 plotline in which jilted nurses boycotted McSteamy's surgeries. Even the Rose plotline that aired in late 2007 and 2008 presented the nurse as wide-eyed about romance with a physician. The pretty Rose was perhaps the only recurring nurse character on *Grey's* who could really be called positive. Rose dated neurosurgeon Derek "McDreamy" Shepherd, but the doe-eyed naïf confessed to being intimidated by the "legend" of the prior romance between Derek and Meredith. In one intensely embarrassing scene in an April 2008 episode, Rose expressed public amazement that she was actually dating the great man: "I'm trying to play it cool. I *am* playing it so, so cool. I love him!"

*House* has not bothered with nurses enough to have as many naughty nurse images as *Grey's*. But a February 2007 episode did invite its 26 million U.S. viewers to chuckle at that irreverent genius House's suggestion that if a physician friend would just stop annoying him, they could be "ranking nurses in order of do-ability." And in a November 2005 episode, the resourceful House coerced a reluctant surgeon into performing a risky liver transplant by threatening to tell his wife what the surgeon had secretly been doing with lots of nurses. Skanky syph nurses, we bet!

An April 2004 episode of the sitcom *Will & Grace* focused on the frivolous Jack character's graduation from "nursing school." At the tiny ceremony, one of the nurse speakers was a very attractive woman whose sheer white uniform was unbuttoned below the level of her bright blue bra. Jack began to read the speech he got to deliver because he was voted "most popular," but decided in the middle that he would follow his original dream of being an actor. Later Will delivered the rest of the speech privately to the blue bra nurse, who was moved by its "follow your dream" theme to muse, "Maybe I will get back into porn."

Beyond prime time, the landscape is hardly better. Even David Letterman, who gave nurses credit following his heart bypass surgery, has been unable to resist the naughty nurse's charms. In December 2005, his CBS *Late Show* included a segment about an injury to his hand. Dr. Robert Hotchkiss, a real hand surgeon, strode out followed by two models dressed as "nurses" in short white dresses and caps. Hotchkiss examined the wound and bantered with Dave. The "nurses" giggled. Preparing for Hotchkiss to remove the stitches, Dave asked if there would be any disrobing. Paul Shaffer interjected, "Just the nurses!" The physician was the witty expert. The "nurses" were sex props.

The naughty nurse has graced other late night shows on a more regular basis. During the 2007–2008 season, USA Network's *Dr.*

*Steve-O* featured *Jackass* veteran Steve Glover "de-wussifying" awkward men by cajoling them into doing painful or embarrassing stunts. At Dr. Steve-O's side throughout was "beautiful hot babe Trishelle," an actress dressed as a naughty nurse. Trishelle's role involved looking cute, letting Steve-O cuddle with her, and encouraging participants to do as Steve-O said. The show was obviously tongue-in-cheek, and viewers no doubt realized Trishelle was not a real nurse, but she still reinforced the stereotype of nurses as peripheral female sex toys.

It's no surprise that the naughty nurse appears on soap operas, which feature a toxic stew of nurse stereotypes, including vacuous handmaidens, gossiping twits, and, uh, monkeys. From 2004 to 2005, the CBS daytime drama *As the World Turns* featured nurse character Julia Larrabee, memorialized in a December 2004 *TV Guide* piece entitled "'Nurse Skank Strikes Again." The character was a "needy, man-hungry nurse" whom fans hated for breaking up some of the soap's most popular couples.

But some might be surprised that the naughty nurse has made notable appearances on supposedly responsible daytime talk shows. In November 2004 psychologist Dr. Phil ran a segment on his syndicated show about the damage a physician had done to his family by having an affair with a nurse. Dr. Phil offered these pearls of wisdom:

> Now, you know, I spent — I spent a lot of years in the health care delivery system, and I watched doctors and nurses play footsie back and forth. And I watched doctors whose wives worked, put them through medical school, all this, and they come up there with a cute little nurse and they start playing footsie with her. I've seen lots of cute little nurses go after doctors, because they're going to seduce and marry them a doctor, because that's their ticket out of having to work as a nurse.

Dr. Phil's statement is a persuasive, insider's vision of nurses as physician gold diggers — the "little" things' bodies are the only way they have to escape their dead-end jobs.

In horror films, the naughty image has often been mixed with malevolence, as in the *Saw III* promotion. You might think nurses are harmless sluts — the conventional view — but in reality, they're forces of evil! Nurses figured in the successful 2006 horror film *Silent Hill*, which was based on popular Konami video games about a haunted town. In the video games, the nurses were monsters, deformed manifestations of human fears who appeared in the game's hospital setting, only occasionally presenting sexually. In the film they were provocatively dressed and ended up blindly killing each other — capturing the effect of naughty nurses pretty well. The 2006 film *Candy Stripers* — not to be confused with the Roger Corman-produced 1974 classic *Candy Stripe Nurses* — was about a hospital full of sexy, horny "candy striper nurses" who had been infected with an alien virus, which they spread through...close contact. And *Sick Nurses*, a low-budget 2007 Thai film, featured seven hot nurses as what one review called a "harem" to a young hospital physician who provided cadavers to body-parts dealers. The nurses liked to take most of their clothes off. But when one nurse got a little too jealous of the physician attention another was receiving, a ghostly horror plot developed. Scary!

## Night Shift Nurses: Nursing in Sexually Oriented Products

The naughty nurse often practices her love in products whose purpose is mainly sexual. This includes pornography in all its forms, as well as lingerie and Halloween costumes.

The naughty nurse thrives in hard-core pornography world-wide. In 2008 hundreds of nurse-themed hard-core feature films were available. They included *Lesbian Big Boob Squirting Nurses* (2008), *Asian T-Girl Latex Nurses 4* (2007), *Penthouse Letters Night Nurses* (2006), *Trailer Trash Nurses 7* (2003), *Nasty Backdoor Nurses* (2001), *Student Nurses* (2000), and *Night Shift Nurses* (1987) — this last one is also the title of a popular fetishistic Japanese *hentai* (por-nographic animation) series begun in 2000. Some Internet sites are devoted to hardcore nurse imagery. In 2008 www.mysexynurses.com offered many videos and thousands of photographs. Compa-rable sites included www.hotnakednurses.com, www.filthynurses.com, www.hotnurses.co.uk, and www.linfirmiere.com (the nurse). The images range from female models shedding clothes to multiple actors, including male "doctors," engaging in intercourse and other sex acts. The women wear, or almost wear, skimpy "nurse" outfits or lingerie, usually white — no patterned scrubs here! Hundreds of general porn sites and networks include naughty nurse sections. And it seems that no female porn star's resume is complete without some nurse imagery. Maybe it's like doing Shakespeare is for mainstream Hollywood stars.

The naughty nurse is also popular in less graphic sexually oriented products, including "lad's magazines," newspapers, and Internet mate-rial that may not quite include full nudity. For example, in August 2005, the cover of the Australian magazine *Ralph* featured Gianna, a former contestant on the local *Big Brother* television program, in a bra and panties "nurse" outfit. Gianna made a different naughty nurse outfit a major feature of her time on the reality show. At the end of 2006 and 2007, the *Sun* (UK) — the most widely circulated English-language daily newspaper in the world — ran promotional tie-in pieces for Babes and Boys' naughty nurse calendars. The *Sun* pictorials featured the usual lingerie-nurse outfits, but a key theme was that the models really *were* nurses. One "student nurse" told the *Sun* she posed for "a bit of a laugh" and "a bit of extra money." Plus, "People always joke about nurses looking saucy so it's fun to be the real thing."

The naughty nurse is also poised to spring out of women's closets worldwide. A North Carolina company called 3 Wishes Lingerie has offered a variety of nurse-related items for years. In June 2008 its online selection of more than thirty nurse outfits included the Naughty Nurse, Bad Nurse, Night Nurse, Wet Nurse, Wild Nurse, and our favorite, Head Nurse. Other retailers sell similar items. In January 2005 the Australian Nursing Federation persuaded retailer Bras N Things to end advertising for one "naughty nurse" outfit, though it remained for sale in the lingerie chain's 150+ stores. As of mid-2008, the retailer's website offered a Nurse Feel Good Outfit. And every year at Halloween, major U.S. retailers, including Party City and Costume Express, sell many naughty nurse costumes. Just harmless fun? The Southern Poverty Law Center's highly regarded Teaching Tolerance campaign has urged the public to reconsider stereotypes even in Halloween costumes.

## Promiscuous Girls: The Nurse in Pop Music

The naughty nurse is a bit of a pop music groupie, and she lets musicians use her to sell or accompany their music, even if the music itself makes no mention of nurses. Examples run across musical styles.

Julie Taymor's 2007 film *Across the Universe*, a musical about the upheavals of the 1960s featuring Beatles songs, included a number in which Salma Hayek played a small group of identical "nurses," all wearing a little black nurse's dress. The sexy Hayeks appear in a hospitalized male character's hallucination and help him sing

"Happiness Is a Warm Gun," as they dance around somewhat provocatively. Finally, one Hayek injects the bedridden man with a syringe containing a little blue naked woman. The nurses' main line: "Bang, bang, shoot, shoot!"

In 2005 the UK electronic-alternative-pop duo Goldfrapp set a video for their single "Number 1" at a plastic surgery clinic where everyone but singer Alison Goldfrapp has a human body and a dog's head. In director Dawn Shadforth's video, Goldfrapp acts like a dog, dances with the clinic staff, and spins the song's tale of animalistic sexual obsession. The "nurses" are all females in short dresses who hand things to the all-male "physicians." The camera dwells on the nurses' bottoms — on which the physicians, at one point, playfully place their stethoscopes.

Country rock singer Keith Anderson's song "XXL" (2005) is an ode to the big and tall, and their ability to get hot babes. The song describes the singer's birth: "Took two nurses to hold me and one nurse to slap me." Trey Fanjoy's video features the famously well-endowed Mötley Crüe drummer Tommy Lee as the leering "doctor." Tommy's lab coat says "Dr. Feelgood" (a Crüe song). In the delivery room, he is on intimate terms with three naughty nurses, who pose, pout, and spill out of their tiny dresses — as they all care for the "XXL" infant and his mom. Paging Dr. Freud to OB!

The punkish pop band blink-182's hit 1999 CD *Enema of the State* featured photos of porn star Janine dressed as a nurse. The front cover shows Janine with the front of her white uniform opened to reveal a red bra, as she pulls on a blue examining glove. The back cover has her sitting on a stool dressed in a short naughty nurses' uniform, holding a huge syringe and needle. The band members, facing her, are dressed only in their underwear, looking concerned. In the photos, Janine seems both seductive and threatening — not unlike some recent horror film nurses.

"The Nurse," a song from the White Stripes' 2005 album *Get Behind Me Satan*, offered a more subtle take on the nurse as romantic object. The Detroit garage rock duo's song isn't naughty, but it does use an unholy mix of nursing imagery to complain about betrayal. Songwriter Jack White sings, "The nurse should not be the one who puts salt in your wounds." He also mentions promises this "nurse" has broken, and laments that the "maid that you've hired could never conspire to kill," not wanting to believe it.

White's metaphors compare the faithful care one would expect from a nurse to that of close friend, presumably a female lover. Wouldn't it be tragic if a "nurse," rather than taking care of you, instead hurt you? Yeah, man. Nurses are obligated to protect their patients, but that doesn't mean their expert care is like romance. And a man may need a "maid," as Neil Young once sang, but he isn't getting a "nurse" every time he gets a lover.

## Hot or Not? Sexy Nurses in the News Media

The naughty nurse is a little more reticent about appearing in the news media. But she still pops out of articles about kooky hospital policies, discussions of current issues, and even comic strips.

The mainstream press is always ready to leap on a nurses-and-sex story. It gets the chance when health facilities seem to be either promoting or discouraging naughty nursing. In March 2008 news sources worldwide reported that a clinic in Spain had told its nurses they would be docked pay if they failed to dress in miniskirts. These reports were partly wrong, as the clinic was only requiring the nurses to wear traditional outfits with a modest-length skirt and cap. That was regressive enough. But major news sources worldwide (such as ABC News) gleefully embraced the miniskirt angle.

Similarly, the Ananova Internet news site has aggressively covered efforts by hospitals in Southeast Europe to get unruly nurses back into skirts. In September 2006 the site's "Nurses in Romania to Wear Miniskirts" reported that "doctors" in a Romanian town had asked "officials" to order female nurses and physicians to wear miniskirts, ostensibly because it would be more "elegant." Somehow, the female physicians did not make the headline. In October 2005 the *Hindustan Times* (India) site posted an Ananova-based item reporting that a Croatian hospital had ordered nurses to "go back to wearing skirts instead of trousers after complaints from patients." The hospital director was quoted as noting that the skirts' length, "be they mini skirts or otherwise," was up to the nurses. The *Hindustan Times* ran this lead: "It has long been suspected that pretty nurses doing their 'nightingale' rounds in their freshly-starched skirts, more often than not, bring a cheer to even the most woefully-ill patients, and now it seems that believers in this theory were right all along." The headline: "Patients Want Pretty, Skirt-Clad Nurses!"

On the other hand, in September 2006 the *Daily Mail* (UK) was compelled to report a sad setback for the naughty nurse. "Nurses Face Ban on Thongs and Cleavage" explained that an Essex hospital was considering requiring nurses to make sure they don't expose cleavage or underwear. And in case anyone missed that message, the *Daily Mail* included an image of the Christina Aguilera naughty nurse ad for Skechers, with this caption: "Sorry guys: don't expect to see the likes of Christina Aguilera in this nurses uniform at Southend Hospital."

News media humorists are not above using the naughty nurse to extract cheap laughs. In an April 2008 edition of Fox News Channel's early morning show *Redeye*, host Greg Gutfeld and his guests conducted what amounted to a loving, if ironic, celebration of the

Spanish clinic's misreported "miniskirt" policy. Gutfeld displayed photos of naughty nurse models, then asked his guests, including a physician, who could be against the clinic's miniskirt policy. Guess what? No one was! Gutfeld asked if "attractive nurses in short skirts might lift the spirits of male patients and increase their chances of getting better." Guest Diana Falzone, co-host of *Devore & Diana* on Maxim Sirius radio, replied, "You know what, I believe that. Every woman no matter what size or shape has something to flaunt. Especially the Latina women. They have big butts. So I say, wear the miniskirts and just save some lives."

In June 2007 syndicated radio host Stephanie Miller and sidekick Jim Ward managed to work naughty nurses into a discussion of proposed federal immigration legislation. When a caller suggested that a provision easing restrictions on the entry of foreign nurses would undermine unions, Miller seemed sympathetic but also noted jokingly that "Jim will not be happy if a lot of naughty foreign nurses get in."

> *Ward:* Naughty nurses by the boatload.
>
> *Miller: (with sound effect of a whip cracking)* Jim cannot…no. We must stop the naughty Scandinavian nurses *(whip)*, porn nurse from infiltrating America *(whip)*.
>
> *Ward:* And French maids. Mmm-hmm.

Miller and Ward are playing with the stereotypes, but not questioning them. Like the whip sound, they are just standard comic effects to be exploited — although, even after four decades and thousands of repetitions, that naughty nurse joke is still a *killer*.

Not even the comics page can escape sexy nurses' plans for world media domination. In March 2008 Matt Janz's syndicated *Single and*

*Looking* strip featured a character asking his friend Zoog whether he'd like to live to be a hundred years old. Zoog: "Sure, Sammy... There's something hot about a young nurse giving me a sponge bath." And in December 2006 John McPherson's syndicated *Close to Home* comic showed an ambulance, and an EMT giving a stretcher-bound patient a choice: "Mercy Hospital" was "20 minutes closer," but the nurses at "Saratoga Hospital" were "really hot." A piece by Charles Fiegl in the *Post-Star* of Glen Falls, New York, about nurses' reactions to the strip reported that McPherson had based it on his desire to impress the nurses at the actual nearby Saratoga Hospital. Asked for comment, one nurse from that hospital reportedly said she and her colleagues really were "very hot," which is "how we get our patients to come to Saratoga," though she added that the nurses there "also provide great care."

Whenever a real nurse describes her profession mainly in terms of physical attraction — as hot or not — the naughty nurse smiles. It's time for a penny shot!

# CHAPTER 6

# Who Wants Yesterday's Girl?

I N JUNE 2008, IN WASHINGTON, DC, a female attorney we know described a problem with a friend's preschool age daughter. This poor girl insisted that she wanted to be a *nurse*! Her mother, a PhD married to an MD, PhD, was aghast. She tried valiantly to persuade her daughter that, if she wanted to work in health care, she should do the "feminist" thing and be a physician, like Daddy. Our attorney friend shared the mother's bewilderment.

In April 2008 a Chicago artist was having dinner with two nursing leaders. The artist spoke sadly about the downward trajectory of her daughter's career aspirations. When her daughter was in elementary school, she had wanted to be a *physician*. But in middle school, her daughter decided she wanted to be a *nurse*. The artist's theme was that society still pushes women into traditional pursuits that limit them. She concluded by noting that her daughter had had four kids and become a stay-at-home mom.

Too much of society continues to believe that nursing is not good enough for smart modern women — that it's only for yesterday's girls (we use the diminutive "girls" deliberately). So it's no shock that men who pursue nursing still encounter resistance. In an extensive 2005 survey of men in U.S. nursing, "eighty-two percent noted that nursing is plagued by common misconceptions that emphasize the view that nursing is a female profession dominated by women, that men are not suited to it because they are not caring, and that men in nursing are gay."[1]

In 2000 the ad agency JWT Communications conducted a focus group study of 1,800 school kids in ten U.S. cities that found that when the conversation on careers changed to nursing, the males in the group stopped paying attention, saying that the conversation no longer applied to them.[2] In February 2008 nurse Robert Zavuga published "Check Bias Against Male Nurses" in the *New Vision* (Uganda). Zavuga noted that people call him a "male nurse" as if that were an oddity, different from "nurse." One nurse we know says that when someone remarks that he is a "male nurse," he tells them that he applied to become a "female nurse," but the classes were all full.

The view that nursing is for women with limited options undermines nursing recruitment, retention, and practice. A 2004 survey found that many U.S. high school guidance counselors told bright students that they were "too smart" for nursing and should instead pursue fields like medicine or business.[3] In December 2005 the *New Zealand Herald* ran a piece by Vikki Bland with the hopeful title "Nursing in Terminal Decline." The piece reported that "few secondary school pupils are interested in nursing." Some career advisers view nursing as "less than ideal from a feminist or masculine perspective" and steer promising students away. An adviser tried to talk New Zealand Nurses Organization chief Geoff Annals' own daughter out of pursuing nursing in favor of medicine. Even those who do become nurses have internalized these social attitudes, which continue to disrupt their sense of professional well-being and self-respect: who wants to *be* yesterday's girl?

In the United States, both men and women became more interested in entering nursing in the mid-2000s, as discussed in chapter 1. However, nursing schools lacked the faculty, infrastructure, and other resources they needed to train the students they attracted. A society enduring a weak economy seemed to have gotten the message that nursing had plentiful jobs but not the message that training skilled nurses requires significant resources. In 2006 one U.S. nursing leader noted that a friend had described a wedding at which another guest mentioned that her son wanted to pursue nursing. But, said the woman, her son had been put on a three-year *waiting list for nursing school*. The mother of a future nurse complained, "This is ridiculous. They could train a nurse in six weeks." Such ignorance is commonplace. As chapter 1 explains, the complex scientific work that nurses really do takes years to learn.

A surge in interest from job seekers will not help nursing in the long run if the public still fails to understand that nursing is a serious modern profession for men and women. And new nurses will not stay at the bedside if social contempt continues to result in severe underfunding of their clinical practice.

The mass media continues to reinforce the view that nursing is simply not good enough for an ambitious modern woman. Every major network Hollywood hospital show of recent years has sent that message, particularly the popular *Grey's Anatomy*, on which young female physicians seem to regard the word "nurse" as the greatest insult they could receive. And recent Hollywood films have celebrated promising girls who, unlike their bitter mothers, did not have to settle for the dead-end job of nursing. The news media often conveys similar views, telling women how they can escape traditionally female jobs like nursing and pursue *real* careers.

Yet this same media is more open to men in nursing than might be expected. Even Hollywood has included some surprisingly good portrayals, such as the Belize character in *Angels in America* and the Ben Parker character on *ER* in 2006–2007. Unfortunately, Hollywood's male nurse characters have at times served as vehicles for "feminist" role reversal — hunky modern men whose subordination to female physicians is clear. On *Private Practice*, young nurse Dell works as a clinic *receptionist*. Still, many helpful press stories have detailed the work of men in nursing and efforts to attract men as a way to address the global shortage. On the other hand, some of the recruitment efforts they describe, which strain to assure us that "real men" can be nurses, may actually reinforce harmful gender stereotypes.

Of course, there are social and historical reasons that people associate caregiving professions with women. And neither women nor men should be excluded from careers on the basis of gender. Women should be able to pursue medicine or any other job they want. But too much of the media regards traditionally female jobs like nursing as menial and insignificant, and defines success in terms of the power and status available in some traditionally male jobs. This is a huge part of the unfinished work of feminism: to help society understand and value the important work that women have traditionally done.

## THE WORK FEMINISM FORGOT

Today even media created by women, such as *Grey's Anatomy*, often expresses overt contempt for nursing, seeming to reflect what journalist Suzanne Gordon has called "dress for success" feminism. In the March–April 2004 article "How Hollywood Portrays Nurses" in the nursing journal *Revolution,* Gordon and nurse Ruth Johnson, explain that media feminists, in their rush to embrace traditionally male fields like medicine, have failed to learn the importance and complexity of "caregiving" fields like nursing. As they note, nursing professor Ellen Baer decried the "feminist disdain for nursing" in a February 1991 *New York Times* op-ed piece. Many media feminists treat nurses with the same explicit condescension that women in general once experienced. In some ways, nurses are the new women.

There have been press items describing the work of strong, able women in nursing, including some of the better pieces discussed in chapters 3 and 4. But recent fictional portrayals of nursing as being worthy of a strong woman tend to be focused on the distant past. Joe Wright's 2007 film adaptation of Ian McEwan's 2003 novel *Atonement* suggested that nursing was a way for women to break out of their traditional roles in the World War II era. And Anne Perry's mystery novels about Victorian-era detective William Monk, published from 1990 through at least 2006, feature tough, intelligent nurse Hester Latterly. Latterly, who worked with Florence Nightingale in the Crimea, is far more assertive than some characters think she should be.

In other words, nursing might have been the feminist thing in the 1860s, or even the 1940s. But you've come a long way, baby! You don't have to be a nurse anymore.

## Hollywood Feminism

Major hospital television shows reflexively suggest that women achieve in health care only by pursuing medicine. It is an obvious subtext in *Grey's Anatomy*, *House*, and *Private Practice*, which focus on the professional development of their many female physician characters. Even *ER* and *Scrubs*, which do have one major nurse character each, have spent very little time on the career development of female nurses.

Consider *ER*. A February 2004 *TV Guide* cover story about the show asks us to "consider the increased enrollment of women in medical schools since *ER*'s 1994 debut." The show's physician advisor Fred Einesman notes that "once *ER* went on the air, emergency medicine became the most popular residency and the number of women who applied went up dramatically." In accord with the show creators' pride in promoting female physicians, *ER* has focused closely on the challenges they face, while sending negative messages about nursing as a female career choice. In one priceless scene in an April 2005 episode, intern Abby Lockhart confronted an elderly male patient who seemed to respect only older male physicians. The abusive patient, assuming Lockhart was a nurse, snapped that he did not "want some nurse calling the shots around here." So, did the episode's two female writers — one a physician — have Lockhart mount a spirited defense of nursing, in which she herself spent many years saving lives? Not exactly. Lockhart responded, with measured but clear indignation, "I am not a nurse. I'm a doctor." What might she have said?

- "Today I am practicing as a physician. But as a nurse my opinions about your care options would be just as valuable."

- "You're absolutely right — no nurse or physician should decide what happens to you. That is your right. As it happens, I am a nurse *and* a physician."

- "Ah...I gather you don't like our nurse-centered model of care." (picking up a phone) "Hello, is this Psych?"

- "Don't worry about nurses calling the shots, sir. The nurses only help the patients we want to live."

*Grey's Anatomy* presents a full landscape of female achievement in health care — from new physicians to senior physicians. Nurses represent what women have to settle for if they are not bright and ambitious like the show's physician heroes. Recall the many expressions of contempt for nursing from the show's female interns, including the seething reactions of Meredith Grey and Cristina Yang after intern Alex called Meredith a nurse in the March 2005 premiere, as discussed in chapter 3. The female physicians' priority is not to understand nurses but to distinguish themselves from what they see as an uneducated servant class. Consider the episodes equating nurses' work with grotesque bodily functions, and nurse Rose telling neurosurgeon Derek "McDreamy" Shepherd that she preferred him talking about "boring science stuff" to brooding about a clinical trial. We guess that nutty *science stuff* is just for smart physician girls like Meredith! *Grey's* makes its mean-girl contempt clear in nonclinical portrayals as well. Unlike the female physicians, the nurses are generally not substantial, interesting people. Instead they are ciphers with whom Alex and McSteamy have sex when something is not going right in their relations with the real women who become physicians. That's why, as Cristina remarked about Izzie, "hell hath no fury like a girl whose non-boyfriend screws a nurse," or, to use Izzie's more precise term, a "skanky syph nurse." And though nurse Rose was a positive character in some ways, she was no real competition for Meredith.

Hollywood movies have taken a similar approach. Gordon and Johnson's 2004 *Revolution* article cites Richard LaGravenese's *Living Out Loud* (1998), in which a woman named Judith has dropped out of medical school to marry a medical student. Years later Judith's physician husband leaves her for a younger physician. The film finds the unfulfilled Judith practicing home health nursing. But she finally achieves rebirth in part by returning to medical school. Critics and women's studies scholars saw that as a "feminist" victory.

More recent films have told young females that nursing is a dead-end job that your mother may have ended up with instead of the physician career she wanted, but you can do better. As discussed in chapter 3, *Akeelah and the Bee* falls into this category. The young heroine's mother Tanya tries to keep her daughter focused on schoolwork by citing her own lost opportunities. Tanya shocks Akeelah by telling her that she actually went to college before dropping out and becoming a nurse — evidently, college is not something nurses need. The movie's young achiever message: work hard, fear not, and things like nursing will not happen to you. *Akeelah* also reinforces the idea that persons of color — like women — achieve by joining traditionally esteemed professions, but not by questioning widely shared assumptions about what kind of work has worth.

Similarly, in *Gracie*, the protagonist's mother is an unhappy school nurse who urges her moping daughter to fight to make the soccer team, using her own life as a cautionary tale. Turns out, Mom wanted to be a surgeon! Gracie is incredulous. Her mother explains:

> I wanted to be in the emergency room. So, uh, now I'm a nurse. That's as close as I could get. So if you want to limit yourself, that's fine. But don't let other people do it for you.

Duly motivated by the fear that she might otherwise be condemned to a life of nursing, Gracie fights to realize her dream. Not surprisingly, promotion and reporting on *Gracie* described the mother as having had to "settle" for being a nurse.

Of course, it's not irrational to assume that if an oppressed group is confined to a few specific jobs, none of those jobs is worthwhile. Not irrational; just wrong. Those who "limited" women to jobs like nursing in the past did not necessarily understand the jobs' true nature any better than "feminists" do today. Little did they suspect that nursing is not trivial scut work, but a vital scientific profession whose members save lives and improve outcomes.

## Escaping the Pink Ghetto: The News Media Tells You How!

There certainly have been press pieces about strong modern women in nursing. But we're not aware of any directly suggesting that a nursing career would advance the interests of society as a whole, the female gender, or any particular female as much as a medical career would. On the contrary, some in the news media have suggested that females who want a real modern career avoid nursing—a view that seems particularly common among those who claim to be advancing the interests of women generally.

In December 2005 Carol Kleiman's career column in the *Chicago Tribune* examined how women can escape the "low wages" and "lack of a career path" in the "pink ghetto" of traditionally female jobs, including nursing and teaching, and move into "demanding" "professional" careers like law and accounting. The author and the consultant who is her main source, Jonamay Lambert, seem unaware that a world without skilled nurses and teachers would also lack the lawyers and accountants they value so highly. And if nurses do have too little money or power, is the solution to urge them all to flee, or to improve their wages and working conditions? Obviously, many nurses *have* fled the bedside. And it seems that those responsible for this piece will be thrilled if they can help even more women escape the "ghetto" of nursing. Of course, fewer nurses means more death. But as the noted employment consultant Ebenezer Scrooge once observed, death is a good way to "decrease the surplus population."

In the July 2004 *New Yorker* piece "To Hell with All That," Caitlin Flanagan compares her mother's return to her career in nursing during the author's childhood to the career-versus-home dilemma that many mothers face today. The article shows a general appreciation for what Flanagan's mother's work meant to her, and even gives some sense that her mother's success at nursing school meant something. But it also seems to reflect a lack of understanding or respect for nursing as a profession.

> It's even harder today than it was in my mother's era, because the modern professional-class mother is not pursuing the kind of women's work for which my mother and her friends had been trained, and to which they eventually returned: nursing and elementary-school teaching and secretarial work and the like. These were posts that could be abandoned and returned to without a significant loss of stature, and were usually predictable in terms of both hours and workload.... Today's career moms are often trying to make partner or become regional sales manager or executive editor, jobs that require a tremendous number of hours and a willingness to allow urgent appeals, via BlackBerry or cell phone, to interrupt even the best-laid plans for family time.

Strictly speaking, Flanagan is comparing jobs decades ago with women's current career options. But readers are likely to come away with their ugliest present-day stereotypes confirmed. In fact, graduate-prepared nurses, including scholars, policy makers, executives, and advanced practice nurses, typically do lose status if they "abandon" their careers. In addition, the nurses who struggle with short-staffing and mandatory overtime would be surprised to hear that their jobs are "predictable" in hours and workload. Flanagan's basic implication is that truly able women today do not do traditional "women's work" like nursing, which is not a "professional career," but a "post" that now rests in the dustbin of smart-girl history.

Nursing also suffers by omission in reports about careers for women. Since former Harvard president Lawrence Summers's negative 2005 remarks about women in science, the media has been full of stories about women's status in "science and engineering" fields. For instance, a long December 2006 piece by Cornelia Dean in the *New York Times* discusses the progress women have made in such fields. This article is more concerned with those who have become university professors in fields like molecular biophysics than it is with the applied sciences or health care. But the piece does note that half of U.S. medical students are now women. And one of the women quoted at length is a New York psychologist. Yet there is not a word about nursing, or the thousands of women with nursing doctorates who are now teaching and conducting scientific nursing research at U.S. universities. Hundreds of thousands have at least a master of science degree in nursing. But in a July 2008 interview with the *Baltimore Sun*, National Organization for Women President Kim Gandy decried the continuing gender segregation in jobs this way: "Why are so few women in STEM careers — science, technology, engineering and mathematics? Those are the careers of the future, where the real money is." In other words, nursing is not a science. And what matters is getting more women into traditionally male fields where the "money" is, not revaluing traditionally female ones like nursing, which are not, evidently, the "careers of the future."

# THE MALE NURSE ACTION FIGURE:
# THE MEDIA CONFRONTS MEN IN NURSING

Men have provided health care to others for thousands of years, but today fewer than 10 percent of nurses worldwide are male. Increasing the number of male nurses is a critical part of helping the profession gain the power and diversity it needs to overcome the current shortage.

The social view that nursing is "women's work" remains strong. Even the English language reflects it. People continue to use "nursing" to mean breastfeeding. The terms "matron" and "ward sister" remain common ones for senior nurses in some nations, including the United Kingdom. Employment specialists use phrases like "pink ghetto," which is not helpful in attracting men to nursing. In 2002 Johns Hopkins University School of Nursing changed its pink student identification cards to green to make men more comfortable wearing them. And many people wrongly believe that all male nurses are gay, or that they're not smart or motivated enough to be physicians, as the NSNA surveys discussed above showed. In view of these attitudes, maybe it's not surprising that a 2003 *NurseWeek* study found that nearly a third of male nurses said they experienced "sexual harassment or a hostile work environment related to the conduct of physicians."[4]

Given this climate, the media's recent treatment of men in nursing could be much worse. Hollywood has had some trouble resisting the male nurse as object of ridicule. Some portrayals have used male nurses for their novelty value, notably for the feminist role reversal described above: nothing makes the new breed of female professionals look more powerful than having a cute male nurse to order around. And in Hollywood portrayals, the sexual identity of male nurses is often an issue in a way it simply would not be for other characters. But even Hollywood has generally resisted the worst stereotypes. The news media has also reported effectively about men practicing nursing, and about efforts to recruit men to help resolve the shortage. These efforts do often stress that "real men" can be nurses, arguably reinforcing exclusionary gender stereotyping, as Thomas Schwarz suggested in his February 2006 piece in the *American Journal of Nursing*, "I Am Not a Male Nurse: Recruiting Efforts May Reinforce a Stereotype."

Some recruiting materials strike a good balance. A clever, irreverent one-minute rap recruiting video created in 2004 by nurse Craig Barton and other ED staff at the University of Alabama at Birmingham shows ED nurses of both genders grinning and strutting toward the camera, as Barton raps about specific, at times technical aspects of the nurses' work. Gender does not seem to be an issue. Another interesting item is Archie McPhee's Male Nurse Action Figure, on sale since 2004. Of course it would have been better to simply call him a "nurse": we can tell he's male. And there is a tongue-in-cheek element, as in other McPhee items. But the product says nothing directly about sexual identity. Instead, the package notes that men who become nurses "are blazing the trail as role models and mentors for generations to come. Thank a male nurse today!"

## Nurses and Murses: Men in Hollywood Nursing

Hollywood has paid considerable attention to men in nursing given that these nurses still make up fewer than 10 percent of the total. Some portrayals have been good, though even some generally helpful ones have had fun with the male nurse stereotype. This has often occurred through juvenile wordplay, like calling someone a "murse" or giving the nurse character a name that suggests a lack of conventional manliness.

Belize, the tough, skilled, imperfect nurse in the film *Angels in America*, is perhaps the best recent Hollywood portrayal of a man in nursing. As explained in chapters 3 and 4, Belize is a 1980s AIDS nurse caring for dying power broker Roy Cohn. The closeted Cohn notes that Belize is his "negation," an openly gay black nurse who will "escort me to the underworld." Cohn lashes out at Belize from the first moment. Yet when Cohn admits to his own need for human contact, Belize is honest with him about his likely fate. He advises Cohn to avoid the radiation the physicians will push on him. When Cohn wonders why he should trust a nurse instead of his "very expensive, very qualified WASP doctor," Belize snaps, "He's not queer. I am." With luck viewers won't think this is the sole reason for Belize's expertise. Belize also advises Cohn, who has pulled strings to get into an early AZT trial, to beware of the "double blind," which may result in his getting a placebo instead of the real drug. Belize is convinced, as many AIDS activists were, that things are moving far too slowly, while thousands die. In his view, he is protecting his patient from a dysfunctional health care and political system.

Perhaps the best-known film portrayals of a man in nursing are in Jay Roach's hugely popular romantic comedies *Meet the Parents* (2000) and *Meet the Fockers* (2004). In late 2008 a third installment of the series was reportedly on the way. In these films, the lead character is "male nurse" Gaylord Focker.

In *Meet the Parents*, Chicago nurse Gaylord, who prefers to be called Greg, faces off with prospective father-in-law-from-hell Jack Byrnes, in an attempt to win Jack's blessing for a marriage proposal to his daughter Pam during a visit to the family's Long Island home. Jack, an intense, WASPy retired CIA agent, turns the visit into an interrogation and son-in-law fitness test for the easygoing, Jewish Greg. Since part of Jack's skepticism about Greg relates to Greg's career choice, common misperceptions of nursing are a recurring theme. Despite condescending challenges to Greg's intellect and manhood from Jack and others, including the physician who is about to marry Jack's other daughter, Greg stands his ground. He refuses to quit nursing despite pressure from Jack. He explains why he became a nurse despite high MCAT scores, why he finds nursing more fulfilling than he would have found medicine, and that nursing is in fact a paid profession, not volunteer work, as Pam's ex-fiancé implies. The character might have done more to rebut the stereotypes, and some men in nursing argued that it would have been better not to present the stereotypes at all. But the stereotypes do exist, and we believe it is useful to examine and reject them, as the film does. Greg's tormentors are generally presented as ignorant and status-obsessed. The film is built around Greg's comic misadventures, but he is a smart, resourceful nurse who endures real adversity to win the woman he loves.

Unfortunately, the sequel *Meet the Fockers* took several steps backward for nursing. Greg has finally earned a place within Jack's "circle of trust," and he will soon be able to marry Jack's daughter Pam, provided that all goes well at a weekend get-together at the home of Greg's touchy-feely parents. Greg remains a positive character. However, the film implies that nursing is for people who are good-hearted but not very ambitious. Greg's father proudly displays a "Wall of Gaylord," which celebrates his son's past achievements — mainly certificates of completion and awards for ninth-place finishes. Greg's parents say they never pushed him too hard, because it was more important that he become a good, loving person. Jack sneers at this celebration of Greg's "mediocrity," noting that competition has been a critical element in keeping America strong. The film is not endorsing Jack's views, but it does regard nursing as a good vehicle to show that the heart matters as much as, or more than, the mind. The stereotype that nursing is for people who are nice but kind of slow is particularly damaging for men, who (like Greg) must often explain what they are doing in nursing.

Television portrayals of men in nursing are similarly mixed. Most of the major Hollywood health care shows have occasionally included male nurse characters. Even *Grey's* has included a few scenes with nurse Tyler, the smug, petty bureaucrat who needs the residents to tell him what to do. At least the show makes no issue of his gender. He's mostly just a bitter serf like any other nurse!

Episodes of *Scrubs* illustrate the range of Hollywood portrayals. Early 2003 episodes featured confident, witty nurse Paul Flowers (yes, a male nurse named Flowers). Female physician Elliot dated Paul, who faced anti-male nurse bigotry from physicians who called him a "murse" who did "women's work." And Elliot struggled with her self-esteem when she belatedly learned that Paul was a nurse, not a physician. As with the Focker character, some felt it would have been better not to portray the slurs. But Paul easily rose above them, and the show made sure viewers knew the stereotypes were stupid.

On the other hand, the ridiculous February 2007 *Scrubs* plotline in which the nasty chief of medicine Bob Kelso became a substitute nurse manager while nurse character Carla was on maternity leave effectively endorsed the same kind of stereotypes. The show mocked Kelso for engaging in girly nurse activities. Kelso gossiped with other nurses and was ordered around by attending Perry Cox, who told him to fetch fresh scrubs and "put on a bra, you're distracting some of the other doctors."

Probably the best television portrayals of men as staff nurses have been on *ER*. Since the 1990s the influential show has included at least one male as a recurring minor nurse character, the straight Malik McGrath and, for a time, the gay Yoshi Takata. Both have been presented as competent. *ER* episodes in late 2006 and early 2007 included traveling nurse character Ben Parker, as discussed in chapter 4. Parker was a love interest for major nurse character Sam Taggart, which was in itself a rare indication that nurses are not just potential physician appendages — we can't recall two nurses dating each other on a recent Hollywood show.

But Parker also seemed designed to present a tough, secure, skilled man in nursing. In a November 2006 episode, a belligerent patient approaches the nurses' station and grabs intern Hope hard by the hair. Nearby nurses and physicians seem stunned, but Parker quickly wrestles the man away. Hope: "Thank goodness for Ben." Physician Pratt, watching Parker subdue the man, notes to resident Barnett, "We just got shown up by a murse." Barnett: "Huh?" Pratt: "A male nurse." Barnett: "That's bad…" But as they continue to watch Parker wrestle the patient, attending Morris notes, "Yeah…he's pretty macho, though, huh?" Later this patient starts spitting at everyone from his gurney in a hallway. Again Ben comes to the rescue, wrapping a neck brace around the patient's face, explaining that the brace is more effective because the patient might bite through a simple mask. Even Barnett is impressed: "Where'd you learn that?" Ben: "Just a little parlor trick I picked up at Savannah General."

Arguably the most interesting television portrayals of men in nursing have been the hunky, evolved straight nurses who report to authoritative female physicians in apparent feminist role reversals. The only regular nurse character on *Strong Medicine* (2000–2006) was nurse midwife Peter Riggs, who acted as a foil to the two female physicians who dominated the show. Peter was übersexual, gorgeous, sensitive, and holistic, yet manly — check his motorcycle! At times

Riggs seemed to operate with some autonomy, counseling and treating patients, but his subservience to the show's physicians was clear. In one episode Riggs confronted a powerful ob-gyn who had performed an unnecessary C-section, resulting in a hysterectomy. But she threatened to have Riggs fired, and Riggs's boss, physician Luisa Delgado, had to save him from the ob-gyn's wrath. In the February 2006 series finale, Riggs did affirm that he would rather be a nurse than a physician, resisting pressure from his girlfriend, resident Kayla Thornton, to go to medical school. She called it his "way out of nursing." The show acknowledged male nurse stereotypes; apparently, Riggs's own mother thought he was gay. But his main function seemed to be to reverse the old paradigm of the powerful male physician surrounded by pretty female nurses.

But with the cute receptionist and would-be midwife Dell Parker, *Private Practice* takes the Peter Riggs formula in full reverse. The show has presented Dell as a nurse without significant skill or experience, and it has also mocked his midwifery studies, as discussed in chapters 3, 4, and 9. Like Riggs, Dell is the evolved yet junior male who serves the powerful female professionals. Unlike Riggs, Dell is an empty vessel, a female empowerment fantasy that will serve only to dissuade men from entering a predominantly female profession in crisis. There are few male midwives in real life, but both Hollywood midwife characters have been men — because they have little to do with reality and everything to do with the superficial "feminist" vision of the media creators.

## I Want to Be a Macho Man: Male Nurses in the News

The news media's recent coverage of men in nursing is perhaps the least bad aspect of the media's overall treatment of nursing. Some pieces have candidly discussed the "male nurse" stigma. A July 2007 profile by Christina Chin in the *Star* (Malaysia) describes the reaction of nursing student Irwin Choo's parents on learning that he wanted to pursue nursing: "His mother wept and his engineer father was dead against it. But their reaction is not uncommon — not many parents would be thrilled that their son has chosen to enter the medical profession as a male nurse!" The reporter asks other male nursing students about the "general perception that male nurses are 'soft' (effeminate)," and that "'male nurse' doesn't exactly reek of the 'cool factor.'" In each case, she elicits confident and rational rebuttals from the students.

Press items that describe the work of men in nursing can be helpful whether or not they stress gender. John Blanton's excellent April 2007 *Wall Street Journal* piece about his experience as a new burn unit nurse, discussed in chapter 3, gave readers a sense of nursing skill and autonomy without making any significant reference to the profession's gender makeup. In June 2006 the *Belfast Telegraph* published Jane Bell's portrait of "alcohol liaison nurse" Gary Doherty. "I'm Not a 'Male Nurse' — I'm a Nurse and Proud of It" uses gender as a hook, but it generally keeps the focus on Doherty's pioneering work handling endemic alcohol-related problems at a north Belfast hospital.

In May 2004 Garry Trudeau's comic strip *Doonesbury* featured U.S. military nurse Lieutenant Chance Lebon. Lebon cared for tough regular character B.D., a soldier who lost part of his leg to a rocket-propelled grenade in Iraq. Lebon handles B.D.'s initial chagrin at having a male "night nurse" by steamrolling through it, guiding B.D. through hospital life, skillfully coordinating B.D.'s interaction with loved ones, and making irreverent comments that remind B.D. that he remains part of the human community. Lebon tells his patient that he will not be much of a challenge, since he has lost "only one limb." The nurse was hoping for a "basket case." B.D. says he was hoping for Ashley Judd as his nurse. When B.D. declines to be set up as a celebrity for the nearby press, despite his civilian status as a college football coach, Lebon marvels that he must put "his pants on one leg at a time." B.D. wonders if that's one from "the nurse's joke manual." Lebon: "Number 14."

Still other pieces discuss efforts to attract more men to the profession to help resolve the shortage. Examples include an optimistic August 2003 segment by Joyce Russell on National Public Radio's *Morning Edition*. The segment reported that gender stereotypes about nurses persist, but that recent recruiting campaigns have stressed both the "masculine" and the more traditional "compassionate" elements of nursing to which men may now be more open. The University of Texas nursing school, advertising at sporting events and in men's magazines, had boosted its male enrollment to 29 percent. And an April 2003 piece by Eve Tahmincioglu in the *New York Times* featured positive quotes from men who switched to nursing from fields ranging from policing to the high-tech industry.

In June 2006 the *Southeast Missourian* ran a revealing piece by Scott Moyers reporting that Southeast Missouri Hospital had held a "guys-only nursing camp" to interest male high school students in the profession. The nurse recruiter who organized the camp said participants were "brave enough to say 'I'm interested in nursing.'" The students shadowed "male nurses" at work. Jared Lacy, seventeen, said he had gotten "a little" grief about wanting to be a nurse, but his "insecurities" faded when he learned about the salary. He added, "To see somebody come in here sick and to help them get healthy again...well, I want to be a part of that." Of course, given peer pressure, few men have gone to nursing school right out of high school. A nurse anesthetist who participated in the camp said he "doesn't worry about telling people what he does." How does he handle it? "I muster my deepest voice and say: 'I'm a nurse.'" However, female nurses don't have to dramatically alter their voice pitch when telling people what they do. Others cited in the report also assure us that you can be a nurse and a "real man" too. How real? Both the reporter and the camp organizer stressed that the participants were athletes. But we heard nothing about their grades.

An August 2005 piece on the New Kerala website implicitly suggested that transnational migration stemming from the nursing shortage itself might help close the gender gap. The story discussed the apparent surge in interest in nursing among the men in the Indian state of Kerala, noting that local males were being lured by the "lucrative nursing options" overseas, with 20 percent of current Indian nursing school graduates going abroad. The article did not discuss the larger context of the nursing shortage.

Some nations may face even deeper issues in recruiting men. A May 2007 Gulfnews.com piece by Nina Muslim discusses efforts to increase the number of men in nursing in the United Arab Emirates, which appears to rely heavily on foreign nurses. The report says that increasing the number of men in nursing is especially important because they do not face the "taboo" on women having physical contact with men in "conservative Muslim" societies. The article reports that there are now almost no male nurses in civilian hospitals because there are few nursing programs "for men." Emirates Nursing Association president Saeed Fadhel says that there is "no stigma" to becoming a male nurse, though the piece suggests there is a broader stigma — for anyone with other options. In any case, if the genders must be separated in training and clinical practice, constructing a strong local nursing profession will be challenging indeed.

And a September 2004 piece by Colleen Kenney in the Nebraska *Lincoln Journal Star* describes one of the more inventive efforts to recruit men to nursing. "Hunky Nurses Pose for Pin-up Calendar" reports that twelve men who are nurses appear (clothed) in a 2005 calendar published by the Nebraska Hospital Association. The goal is "to help get more men into nursing and to show it's a job for a regular guy." The article emphasizes the calendar guys' "male" activities, such as playing football, lifting weights, and shooting turkeys with arrows. One nurse notes that people tend to assume that he is doing a woman's job, that he is gay (a word it seems he can't quite bring himself to utter), or that he is or soon will be a physician. But the piece does not suggest that it's wrong to look down on male nurses who *are* gay or effeminate. Just don't confuse *us* with *them*.

These efforts point up a dilemma in nursing's issues with gender. There is a huge incentive to address the shortage by any means necessary, even if that means cutting some corners, including in how we sell the profession to the public. Nurse recruiting efforts might tell people it's OK for men to be nurses, whether they fit traditional notions of masculinity or not. But what would the result be if an ad said something like this:

*Gay male nurse:* Some of us are gay.

*Straight male nurse:* Some of us aren't.

*Female nurse:* Whatever...What we all have in common —

*Gay male nurse:* Is that we save lives, and improve patient health every day —

*Straight male nurse:* In a challenging modern scientific career. So —

*Female nurse:* Do you have what it takes to be a nurse?

Can nursing persuade the public to reconsider its assumptions not only about what work matters, but about who men and women are? Maybe it can — if we put our pants on one leg at a time, and muster our deepest voice.

# CHAPTER 7

# You Are My Angel

ONE NIGHT IN THE LATE 1980S, we were at a party on DC's Capitol Hill. A female law student, meeting a nurse friend of ours for the first time, asked what the nurse did for a living. Upon learning the answer, the law student brightened and replied, "Isn't that sweet! That's what I wanted to be when I was in kindergarten!"

The nurse — who had worked all the previous night using her bachelor of science degree to save sick children's lives — was amused.

Two decades later, nurses are still widely regarded as angels of mercy, noble spiritual beings, or loving mothers. The *New York Times*'s annual "Tribute to Nurses" includes real stories, but the advertising supplement promotes them with a focus on touching, feeling, and warming hearts. When television psychologist Dr. Phil tried to make amends for his nurse-as-gold-digger comments, his praise for nursing relied largely on soft helping imagery.

Compassion and caring are important parts of nursing. But the extreme emphasis on "angel" qualities reinforces the prevailing sense that nurses are all about touching and feeling rather than thinking, using advanced skills, or saving lives. It suggests that nurses, as virtuous spiritual beings, have little need for clinical resources, education, rest, or security. The angel stereotype deters men and women (consider that law student) from entering the profession. It implies that nurses should meet certain moral and sexual standards that are not a proper part of the modern workplace. And it is another in the matched set of feminine stereotypes that plague nursing, along with the naughty nurse and the battle-axe. Collect them all! Nursing has.

The angel image is not just something society has forced on nurses. Many nurses and their supporters continue to embrace and perpetuate it. Johnson & Johnson's Campaign for Nursing's Future, which aims to address the nursing shortage, has run sentimental television ads about "the importance of a nurse's touch," though it is unlikely the nursing crisis has occurred because the public forgot that aspect of nursing. Nurses had input on the ads, and many nurses have defended them. Similarly, many stories that nurses present to the public about their work rely heavily on emotional themes, as in popular books like *Chicken Soup for the Nurse's Soul* (2001). These stories have value, but they can also feed the angel stereotype.

Of course, the angel image has deep roots. Nursing was traditionally seen as a religious vocation, and the perception of moral purity gave women social license to provide the intimate care nursing requires. That care requires great strength and inspires genuine appreciation. But the "virtue script" now operates not only to exclude nursing from consideration as a serious modern profession but also to discourage nurses from advocating for themselves — and their patients. Like Jacob in the Bible, nurses must wrestle and overcome the angel.

## WHAT'S WRONG, ANGEL?

The angel image of nursing pleases some, but it has fatal flaws.

The image fails to convey the college-level knowledge base, critical thinking skills, and hard work required to be a nurse. If nurses are angels, then perhaps they can care for an unlimited number of patients, though research shows fewer nurses means higher patient mortality. Maybe nurses can endure inordinate levels of workplace stress and abuse from patients and colleagues, as recent research suggests they do. Maybe nurses can work mandatory overtime, because they don't have children at home needing care, food, or clothing. Angels don't need rent money; they live in heaven. Angels don't eat or go to the bathroom, so they can work thirteen-hour shifts without even a moment's break, as many nurses must do today. The stereotype suggests that nurses are loving nurturers who need no say in health care decision-making or policy. If nurses suffer in such conditions, some may view it only as evidence of nurses' virtue, not a reason to alter the conditions. Likewise, it may be unclear why angels need well-paid professors or years of college-level education: after all, they're mostly just holding hands and lifting spirits.

In everyday conversation, it is more common for women than men to be described as angels. This fact may discourage men from entering nursing. The angel and related maternal stereotypes also complement the "naughty nurse" and the repressed battle-axe images. All define nurses by dubious visions of female sexual extremes, from madonna to whore, rather than by nurses' professional skills or effort. Indeed, some feel that putting nurses in these boxes is a way for vulnerable male patients to reassert their traditional power over the females who now appear to control their lives in the hospital.

In the popular imagination, angels are pure and gentle. But patient advocacy may require that nurses assertively challenge an established system or proposed course of action. Florence Nightingale was no "angel." She was a bright, aggressive, flawed human being who made lasting scientific and social contributions. Good nurses continue that tradition.

In Buresh and Gordon's *From Silence to Voice* and in Gordon's *Nursing Against the Odds* (2005), the authors document the roots, nature, and effects of what they call the "virtue script" of nursing, as we explained in chapter 1. The authors show how nineteenth-century reformers created a respectable job for women by using this moral script and assuring physicians that nurses were no threat to them. Indeed, nurses' historic oppression by physicians parallels the oppression of women by men. The authors argue that because of nurses' socialization in the virtue script and the imperative to "say little and do much," most nurses still display a bone-deep self-effacement and fear of controversy. Even many nursing scholars, Buresh and Gordon note, define the profession mainly in bland relational terms. Angel imagery buries nurses' real knowledge and skill, and this may suit some physicians, who receive the credit and resources nursing would otherwise claim. But the authors argue that nurses must overcome their fears and stop disrupting their own "definitional claims" by reinforcing stereotypes.

We sometimes hear that leaving the angel behind would mean abandoning compassion in nursing, and that that special quality is what sets nurses apart. We agree that nurses must be compassionate. But when nursing is described mainly in terms of female love and devotion, the public views nursing in those terms — not as the work of highly skilled professionals of both genders, but as the work of nuns, or a kind of paid mothering service. Of course, the emotional support nurses give is actually psychosocial care shaped by their training and experience. It does have real health benefits, and it is not something that just any nice person could do.

We think what sets nursing apart is the *combination* of technical prowess, psychosocial skills, and mental toughness nurses use to save lives. But the media tends to ignore the "harder" aspects of nursing, such as nurses' advanced skills and the stress they endure. Gordon notes that while she values nurses' emotional support, if given a choice between a compassionate nurse and one who could save her life, she would take the life saver. The public must understand this life-saving side of nursing in order for the current crisis to be solved.

Nursing has topped the Gallup public opinion poll measuring the "honesty and ethical standards" of different professions every year since nursing was added to the poll in 1999, except in 2001 when firefighters led the list following the 9/11 tragedy. These results go hand in hand with the prevailing vision of nurses as devoted and angelic. But if everyone loves nurses so much, why has a global shortage rooted in a lack of resources and understanding been taking lives worldwide since 1998? Because, we think, what these polls measure has little to do with the real respect that determines how scarce economic and social resources are allocated. Yet even some nursing leaders have embraced the "honest and ethical" label as a reason that policy makers should address nurses' concerns. It seems to us that patients trust nurses to hold their wallets while they're in surgery but not to save their lives. Some professions near the bottom of the Gallup list — such as law and advertising — do not seem to lack willing workers, good working conditions, or social status. And we wonder how many of the people who trust nurses so much would react if their child announced that he or she wanted to be a nurse.

In July 2004 the *American Journal of Nursing* published an op-ed by Margaret Belcher, RN, BSN, entitled "I'm No Angel: I Am a Nurse — and That's Enough." Belcher wrote that while nurses liked imagery focusing on compassion, such imagery did not make her proud. She argued that the emphasis on self-sacrifice has led to "burnout and compassion fatigue." With unusual courage and insight, Belcher got to the heart of the "angel myth":

> I have the education and experience to do for others what they cannot do for themselves. But it's the intimacy of the work that feeds the angel myth. I listen to patients, touch them, reassure them, help them eat and drink, assist them with bodily functions. They are often ashamed of their need for help, and they're grateful to be treated with respect....I don't exist on a higher plane because I work at the bedside....But to call nursing a job rather than a calling isn't to diminish it. I will not stop touching lives if I refuse to call the work magic. I will not be a failure if I give up self-sacrifice for self-care. Nurses have not learned this lesson well. If we indeed were to put ourselves first, perhaps there wouldn't be a nursing shortage.

As we often hear on airplane flights, we must put on our own oxygen masks before we can help others.

Many "angel" comments from patients and families seem to result from the nurse's cleaning up poop in a way that preserves the patient's dignity. Responding to unpleasant tasks and patient abuse with control and respect may encourage people to call nurses angels. But attributing this difficult work to spiritual grace does the humans who actually perform it a disservice. At the same time, nurses are rarely called angels for detecting a deadly symptom or advocating for a life-saving intervention.

The March 2008 UPI item "Half of U.S. Nurses Bullied on the Job" highlighted yet another study on the high level of abuse nurses face. Research often points to institutional reluctance to address such abuse. Nurses commonly receive inadequate support. Of course, violence against women in general is often discounted. But nurses in particular may be expected to simply "get over it" because they are spiritual beings with a vocation who do not suffer like others do. Angels don't get PTSD.

As Belcher noted, there remains plenty of support for the angel within nursing. A December 2007 editorial in the popular *RN* magazine urged nurses to "put an end to angel bashing." The author asserted that the image arose from nurses' helpful behavior with patients, and getting rid of the image would require that nurses stop being helpful. Some responding letters reflected the views that the angel is better than some of the alternatives and that jettisoning the image would require moving to the other extreme. Nurses would lose their focus on "caring" and become harsh technicians. However, the nursing image need not be confined to stereotypical extremes. We believe that the public is capable of seeing nurses as three-dimensional beings: strong, skilled professionals of both genders who excel at both technical tasks and the psychosocial work often described as "caring" and "compassion."

## BLESS THIS ANGEL OF MERCY NURSE COLLECTIBLE FIGURINE!

Angel imagery continues to infect the media's treatment of nursing. These images range from casual references to in-depth portrayals, from daytime television to the print press. Let's look at some notable examples.

## Angels Everywhere

For some media sources, the word "angel" is interchangeable with "nurse." In January 2007 the *Scotsman* ran Angus Howarth's "Robot Nurses Could Be on the Wards in Three Years, Say Scientists." The piece reported that the "mechanised 'angels'" would "perform basic tasks such as mopping up spillages, taking messages and guiding visitors to hospital beds." These "angels" aren't exactly working at the core of patient care, are they? In January 2005 the *Guardian* (UK) website posted Jamie Doward's "Row Erupts over Secret Filming of Hospital Filth," about a television documentary for which two nurses used hidden cameras to document "appalling conditions" at two British hospitals. The documentary was named *Dispatches: Undercover Angels*.

Television personality Dr. Phil tried several times to make amends for his 2004 comments suggesting that many nurses were out to marry physicians in order to avoid "having to work as a nurse," which we discussed in chapters 3 and 5. In a December 2004 statement he assured viewers that the "men and women" in nursing are "dedicated," "devoted," "extremely well-trained," and "the backbone of the medical profession." He also noted that no matter "how much technological advance we make with machines to monitor patients, machines can't do the loving, nurturing care that a nurse can do, can't have the judgment, can't have the wisdom and can't be replaced by machines." Machines do help nurses assess patients and plan care. But Dr. Phil's statement suggests that maybe technology really does do everything except for nurses' angelic "loving" and "nurturing." More broadly, most of his comments paint nursing as a physically demanding support vocation focused on emotional care. The "backbone" is important, and apparently even "loving," but it doesn't do any thinking.

In April 2005 Dr. Phil's show aired "Stories of Survival," which featured two victims of "senseless" violence who were living with permanent facial disfigurement. They were a former deputy sheriff named Jason and Dr. Phil's sister-in-law Cindi Broaddus. The idea seemed to be to help Jason and his family, using Cindi as an inspirational example. Another guest was nursing assistant Daphne, who had helped Cindi during her recovery. Dr. Phil, Cindi, and Clarice Marsh, director of pediatric nursing at UCLA, offered brief testimonials for nursing as the underappreciated "backbone" of health care, as Dr. Phil again put it.

The episode mostly suggested that nurses are virtuous, hardworking hand-holders. Marsh did say that nurses are "incredibly intelligent" and that their work is "multi-faceted." She also said that in nursing "the art is the relationship," and that nurses form a "bond" that can't be found anywhere else. Dr. Phil said Daphne was a "wonderful example" of this. Yet nursing assistants, who have minimal training, are not nurses. Dr. Phil said he did not think Cindi would have made it without the "tremendously inspired and dedicated" nursing staff. Cindi agreed that nurses were "wonderful, wonderful." But no one said what nurses actually *do*. During her four minutes of screen time, Daphne did not utter *one word* that was audible to viewers. The last shot in the segment was a close-up of the nursing assistant and Cindi holding hands. We commend Marsh for her positive general statements, but the comments about the nurse-patient "bond" and the "art of the relationship" — with nothing concrete about nurses' clinical skills — are consistent with the overall angel impression.

The *New York Times* publishes an annual "Tribute to Nurses." To gather the stories it includes, the paper uses language like this, from April 2007:

*The New York Times* invites you to share your personal story in The Nursing Diaries. Whether heartwarming or humorous, we want to know your inspirations, challenges, lessons learned and experiences that have left a footprint on your heart forever.

A *footprint*? Despite this (presumably unintentional) nod to the stress of nursing, the stories that the *Times* collects with this kind of language tend to reinforce the sense of nurses as virtuous angels rather than life savers. Note the paper's use of the word "heart" twice in a single sentence.

In September 2006 the *Liberty Times* (Taiwan) profiled Chuan Ya-lan, a young nurse who "has become lauded by the Taichung Hospital as an angel for her service." Chuan "exhibits an extraordinary degree of patience with the patients, and everyone comments how nice she is." Indeed, Chuan is "a model in terms of having the compassion and expertise required of a nurse." A manager says many new graduates cannot cope with the "heavy workload and stress" of handling at least eight patients at a time, and most "resign after a relatively short period." But Chuan has "never complained about the workload." This piece certainly offers a positive view of Chuan. But its "angel" focus (despite the passing reference to "expertise") says that nurses are relatively unskilled spiritual beings who can be expected to make inhuman sacrifices. We might see a willingness to assume an enormous patient load without complaint as laudable devotion — or as a sign that nursing is too weak to stand up for itself or its patients. A nurse may be able to endure a patient load of eight or more, but as research shows, her patients cannot.

In June 2005 the *Age* (Melbourne) ran "Saint Be Praised," Brian Courtis's profile of actress Georgie Parker and her television character, a nursing manager on the popular Australian hospital drama *All Saints*. One good passage suggested that television's heroic health worker narrative may actually undermine efforts to ensure adequate health care funding, but the piece reinforced stereotypes that have the same effect. Parker, the "saintly practitioner of the blessed art of medical melodrama," was leaving *All Saints* after years of "compassionate caring" as "much-loved nurse Terri Sullivan." The character's "enigmatic, soulful and spiritual bedside manner produced miracles" for patients. "Critics loved her, and now network beatification must surely follow." (In fact, beatification is one step toward sainthood; canonization is the actual making of the saint. There's a whole course on this in nursing school.) The report concluded that "St. Terri" had earned her place in the "stained-glass windows of soap opera."

In February 2005 Tickle, the "leading interpersonal media company," offered an online test called "Who's Your Inner Nurse?" The lighthearted test offered respondents a series of stereotypes. One question invited nurses to report that patients found them either gentle, cheerful, dependable, or selfless. We guess there wasn't quite enough room for "expert" or "savvy." Another question gave test takers the chance to specify that they wouldn't "make [their] rounds without" their "stickers and lollipops."

And speaking of lollipops, in March 2008 an Angela Moore jewelry catalog featured Nurse Nancy bracelets composed of four different types of balls strung together. The balls showed a smiling nurse in a white uniform giving a balloon to a girl, a ladybug next to a stethoscope, a nurse's cap with a thermometer, and a stuffed bear holding flowers next to a lollipop. The text asked readers to buy the jewelry to "celebrate the ladies who give lollipops and band aids a whole new meaning."

But that's nothing. For years, companies like Precious Moments have offered figurines that present nurses as noble, selfless, sweet, tender, loving, wonderful, maternal, faithful, special, devoted, cuddly, comforting, gentle, delicate, blessed, adorable saints. And those are the edgy ones. In late 2004 the marketing copy for Precious Moments' Nurses are Angels of Mercy Collectible Figurine revealed that this "adorable" figurine is "ready to flutter into your life on little angel wings; her impish smile and bright eyes are sure to warm your heart." The Bless This Angel of Mercy Nurse Collectible Figurine may be just the thing for the "special nurse" who has given you "comforting attention and care." As for the Special Delivery Nurse Figurine, a teddy bear nurse holding a teddy bear newborn:

> Faithful Fuzzies Nurse is "Beary" Special...No matter how long her shift is, you won't hear this faithful nurse complain, because cradling this little miracle in her arms is reward enough for her sincere devotion. That's because her job requires the "gentle art of caring" — it's more than hard work, it's "heart" work!

This is the virtue script in full bloom: this "nurse" has no complaints no matter how bad conditions are. And the Sending Love from Above Figurine nurse dispenses a "dose of 'loving, caring and sharing'" wherever she goes, from her "delicate angel wings" to her "adorable nurse's bag filled with pink pearlized heart-shaped messages of faith and love." As of 2008 Precious Moments was still selling products along these same lines.

Don't get us wrong: we don't object to this imagery in isolation any more than we do to sexual imagery. Fusing it with the profession of nursing is the problem.

## Nurse or Mom?

Some press items present the nurse as professional mother, no matter how skilled or authoritative she may be, or how good the story may otherwise be. In October 2007 *Time* magazine profiled U.S. Navy Commander Maureen Pennington, the "first nurse to lead a surgical company during combat operations." Caroline Kennedy's "Beyond the Call of Duty" highlights Pennington's leadership, communication, and cross-cultural skills. But even so, the piece focuses on vague helping imagery. A physician's assistant says Pennington was "like a mom to all of us." Pennington herself says she understands Marines: "Being a mother, I know you also have to be willing to be hated in order to be loved. I knew it was up to me to make sure that there were rules and structures in place because people need those too when the world is falling apart." OK, but even a tough, able mother does not necessarily have Pennington's advanced science training and clinical skills. And though we hear all about what kind of mom Pennington is, there is nothing in the story about her education. In fact, she has a master's degree in nursing.

Similarly, in January 2006 the *Detroit Free Press* ran a generally good story by Patricia Anstett about Wayne State University nurse practitioner Mary White. Although the piece focuses on White's innovative methods, which include health-oriented *Jeopardy!* contests and "condom bingo" in the dormitories, it unfortunately also notes that White is "a nurse first and foremost, with all the loving compassion the term typically conveys." Yuck. Later we're told that White is "all pro, plus surrogate mom." One sophomore refers to White as "like a mom to me now." White herself describes her appeal to the students this way: "I'm the mom image, but I'm safe because I don't lecture them." But Mom does not know how to titrate life-saving medications, and Mom is not hosting condom bingo.

## The Fallen Angels

The media also takes an intense interest when nurses *fail* to be noble angels, when they are seen as too demanding or uppity, when they're promiscuous or irreverent, or when they're malevolent "angels of death." Despite the obvious differences, in all of these cases nurses have failed to follow the virtue script.

### THE STRIVERS WHO HAVE FORGOTTEN THEIR PLACE

Some nurses seem to misplace their heart-shaped messages of faith and love. In summer 2006 anonymous UK physicians published op-eds designed to discourage the government from allowing nurses to move into clinical roles that have traditionally been the province of physicians. "Are Nurses Angels? I Don't Think So" ran in the *Daily Mail*, and "Why Nurses Are No Angels" appeared in the *Independent* and the *Belfast Telegraph*. These paternalistic essays urged the National Health Service (NHS) to stop assigning nurses new roles, a practice that had supposedly produced nurses who were stupid, uncaring, lazy, and eager to dump everything on physicians while wrongly seeking the same high status. Instead, the pieces argued, nurses should focus on the basic caring and hygiene tasks the physicians think define nursing. Maybe their halos will reappear.

Christie Blatchford's column "Militant Angels of Mercy," in a June 2003 edition of Canada's *National Post,* yearned for the days when nurses were "kind" and "loved, if not always respected." Blatchford claimed nurses had not received much public support for their work battling SARS because too many had become "outright shiftless or worse, just plain mean." One problem was that nursing had "come to be deemed a capital-P profession, as opposed to a calling," so that people became nurses as much for "opportunities or pay or perquisites" as to help the ill. Maybe Blatchford would rather have a system in which patients perish because the nurses are angelic but unskilled volunteers: at least we'd die smiling! Blatchford links the alleged decline in nursing care to nursing militancy. But she fails to reconcile this self-seeking militancy with the current nursing crisis, which includes a global shortage and often atrocious working conditions.

## PROMISCUOUS GIRLS

Needless to say, nurses may also fall from grace through sex and drugs. Thus, if someone were to create a television series about hot young female nurses hooking up, it might be called *No Angels*.

Oh wait — that actually happened. In February 2004 the *Times* (UK) published nurse Vici Hoban's piece about the new Channel 4 drama called *No Angels*. The show had aimed to "explode the myth of angels by the bedside" and provide "a witty and truthful exposé of nursing" in the modern NHS. But the first episode showed the nurses "laughing over a corpse that they have warmed up in the bath to disguise the fact that the patient died, unnoticed, hours earlier," as well as "tricking colleagues into taking drugs, showing off visible panty lines to doctors and having sex in cupboards." In September 2004 Reuters reported that *No Angels* was "up for translation into a Stateside version," but that has yet to appear. The British show lasted three seasons.

## THE ANGEL OF DEATH

Sadly, as in any profession of millions, there are a very small number of dangerously troubled nurses. Not surprisingly, coverage of their bad acts tends to highlight their deviation from the virtue script.

In November 2004 *Reader's Digest* ran Max Alexander's generally fair cover story on Charles Cullen, a nurse who pled guilty in New Jersey to having killed thirteen patients with drug overdoses, and who by his own account may have killed twenty-seven more. Cullen was shown to have a history of troubled relationships, mental illness, and substance abuse. Unfortunately, the headline was "The Killer Nurse," and the internal subhead was "Why No One Stopped the Angel of Death." Of course, the contrast between the usual angel stereotype and Cullen's actions makes for a great story.

The Cullen story appears to have inspired a December 2004 episode of NBC's short-lived prime-time show *Medical Investigation*, a drama that followed a team led by heroic National Institutes of Health physicians. The show generally presented nurses as peripheral handmaidens, but they finally got some attention in "The Unclean." In that episode, after suspicious deaths at a Baltimore hospital, the investigators search for infection control problems. They finally realize that some "angel of death" has been infecting patients with a bloody sheet. They are initially suspicious of a weasely nurse, but he turns out to have been the whistle-blower (though he gets no credit). The team ultimately finds that the "angel of death" is in fact a meek, helpful nurse who has gained access to experimental bacteria and, like the real-life Cullen, has left a trail of suspicious patient deaths at her prior jobs. The show does not bother to explore why she might have done it.

That reticence is missing from an astonishing April 2004 op-ed in the *Philadelphia Inquirer*. In "Nursing Compassion to Health," NYU forensic psychiatrist Michael Welner actually argues that Cullen's murders were the result of the modern emphasis on "material" benefits in the training and hiring of hospital workers. To reverse this trend, health care facilities should "focus on hiring those with the most compassionate personalities." Apparently Cullen was not an aberrant sociopath, but just an extreme example of what nurses have become.

> Employment ads solicit health-care workers based on material benefits. Whom, then, will such ads aim to attract? Not the nuns of yesteryear....So we need to integrate vigorous empathy training and stress management into medical and nursing education....Tomorrow's professionals need to be prepared for the adverse climate of providing health-care services within institutional frameworks that are insensitive by design.

So the answer to "insensitive" care systems lies not in restructuring health care financing or better oversight, but simply in hiring nicer people with better stress management skills! Nurses are spiritual beings who don't need the substantive training and resources on which other professions rely to ensure high performance. Welner's emphasis on selflessness in health care recruiting did not appear to extend to his own lucrative New York consulting practice, the Forensic Panel. The Panel's website extolled the advanced credentials of Welner and the other consultants, and one of its FAQs addressed the vexing question "How can I afford the services of the Forensic Panel?"

## The Angel Within

Arguably the most striking angel imagery appears in statements by nurses and their advocates. Perhaps it's not surprising that non-nurses who want to express support for nurses conceive of the profession in these terms. Thus, in a February 2008 article in the *Chronicle Herald* (Nova Scotia), "Let 'Angels' Spend More Time Nursing," a grateful cancer patient said his nurses were "the closest I have ever met to angels." And in a June 2007 article from Boston's State House News Service, "Nurses Demand Stronger Protections Against On-the-Job Violence," the husband of a nurse who had been assaulted referred to nurses as "angels in scrubs."

But nurses themselves also continue to embrace the angel. Every year in May, nurses around the world celebrate Nurses Week or Nurses Day. Different organizations have different themes. Some have emphasized nurses' substantive achievements, such as the Geneva-based International Council of Nurses (ICN) with its "Safe Staffing Saves Lives" (2006) and "Delivering Quality, Serving Communities: Nurses Leading Primary Care" (2008). However, from 2000 to 2002, each ICN theme included the emotional phrase "Always there for you." The American Nurses Association (ANA) adopted as its 2000 theme the angel-tastic "Nurses: Lifting Spirits, Touching Lives." In 2004 the ANA's "Nurses: Keeping the Care in Health Care" implied that nurses focus on "care" while someone else (guess who!) takes the lead on "health." Even the group's vague 2008 theme, "Nurses: Making a Difference Every Day," fits with the idea that nurses are all about intangible uplift.

Perhaps most ironic is the tendency of media aimed directly at resolving the nursing shortage or recruiting nurses to use angel imagery, particularly when that seems to serve a larger institutional interest. In 2002 Johnson & Johnson initiated the massive Campaign for Nursing's Future to address the nursing shortage and increase interest in nursing careers. The company financed an extensive nursing website, raised funds for faculty fellowships and student scholarships, and sponsored the helpful 2004 recruiting video *Nurse Scientists: Committed to the Public Trust.*

But the J&J campaign project with the greatest influence was undoubtedly the television ads. The theme of the early ads was "the importance of a nurse's touch." The spots included a few elements suggesting that nurses had some skill, and the caring young nurses who appeared were diverse. But the soft-focus ads relied mainly on angel and maternal imagery. The three spots that began airing in 2005 all featured the same semi-cooing female narrator, the kind of voice used to advertise cuddly products for babies. The opening: "At Johnson & Johnson, we understand the importance of a nurse's touch." The closing: "Nurses: we need you more than ever. A message of caring from Johnson & Johnson." One ad used the word "touch" five times in thirty seconds. The focus on "caring" and "touching" nursing images clearly serves the business interests of a major pharmaceutical company. J&J has long projected a baby soft image, and fusing that image with the nursing angel stereotype reinforces the idea that the company is as honest and ethical as nurses are seen to be. But these images do nursing no favors.

In 2007 J&J unveiled two new spots. These did not abandon angel imagery, particularly in the use of gooey music with lyrics about being "born to care," which suggests that nursing is more of a divine vocation than a profession requiring intensive training. But both ads did emphasize that nurses are not just angelic hand-holders. They made clear that nurses save lives and improve outcomes, even offering specific examples, like defibrillation. One ad paid tribute to nurse educators, showing the impact they have through their students.

In 2007 the University of Michigan ran radio ads featuring men describing why they became nurses at the university. The ads seemed to be directed at recruiting nurses and nursing students, though they may also have been part of the university's capital campaign. The nurses came off as substantial people whose work has real meaning.

Sadly, the ads relied on generalized, emotional angel imagery. We heard about the nurses setting up a summer camp for disabled kids, getting smiles, loving what they do and not looking at it as a "job," "helping" kids fight cancer, inspiring and being inspired. But nowhere did listeners hear what nurses *actually do for patients.* The virtue script message the ads sent was, at best, uninspired.

## TRANSCENDING THE ANGEL: WHAT CAN BE DONE?

Because angel imagery is so deeply embedded both in the public consciousness and nursing culture, overcoming it will be a challenge. But it can be done. Nurses can have a public image that acknowledges the value of caring and compassion, but that also shows respect for nursing as a skilled modern profession. Any of the media items discussed elsewhere in this book that present nurses as educated, life-saving professionals counter the angel stereotype. As we've seen, HBO's film *Angels in America* actually subverts the most damaging nursing stereotypes.

In May 2005 the California Nurses Association (CNA) vowed to celebrate Florence Nightingale's birthday by staging a protest at the San Francisco offices of Johnson & Johnson. CNA's press release argued that the company had supported recent efforts to limit the political participation of nurses and other public employees, and that it had donated huge sums to defeat measures designed to lower drug prices in California. The union said its protest honored the "legacy of the original nurse activist." Whatever the merits of CNA's specific position, its protest contradicted the inaccurate image of Nightingale and the nurses who have followed her as cuddly saints.

In October 2006 the *Boston Globe* posted a poll on its website after a successful nurses' strike in Worcester. As we noted in chapter 3, the text described contracts under which the "average nurse... working a 40-hour week makes $107,000 a year," and the poll asked whether the nurses "deserve this six-figure salary for what they do." The nurses' union, the Massachusetts Nurses Association, urged nurses to respond to the poll by explaining why they were worth the money. The union reminded nurses, "You work in one of the most dangerous professions (you're injured as much as construction workers, you're assaulted more than prison guards), you deal with deadly infectious diseases; you hold life and death in your hands every minute of every shift."

The Los Angeles poetry magazine *Rattle* placed a "Tribute to Nurses" in its Winter 2007 issue. The forty-five-page section included only nurses' own work. You might think the "tribute" approach would lead editors right to the angel image, but *Rattle* offered insightful essays and well-crafted, irreverent poems that captured modern lives and deaths without sentiment. The poems suggested the scope of patients' lives through their physicality, their frailties, their suffering. To some extent we also saw nurses' complex, sometimes difficult inner lives. The tribute presented nurses not as angels but as keen observers and courageous workers who help us in our darkest hours.

And in 2004 Craig Barton, RN, and other ED staff at the University of Alabama at Birmingham created an irreverent one-minute rap recruiting video. The video is a clever and infectious slice of the life of an urban ED nurse. ED nurses move toward the camera, strutting and grinning, as Barton raps about their work. We hear about starting IVs, and handling a heart patient with a "positive history" who needs "a twelve-lead EKG." More lyrics: "Ka-boom! We're the UAB emergency room! And we treat every single patient from the womb to the tomb!"; "We're ER nurses! Medications we disburses!"; "We expect the unexpected! That's why we're well-respected!"; and "Yo, we're savin' lives up in here!" Barton's engaging focus on nurses' life-saving, technical skill, and team spirit is a welcome alternative to the angel. This one keeps it real.

# CHAPTER 8

# Winning the Battle-Axe, Losing the War

NURSE LINDA S. SMITH once entered the room of a young male inpatient to give him his meds. The patient "grinned and naughtily paraphrased the words he had just read on one of his [get-well] cards: 'Nurse, are you coming in to give me one of those famous sponge baths? If you are, I'm ready!'" On his nightstand, one card showed a sexy young nurse offering sponge services. That much is hardly news — just another hostile work environment linked to the naughty nurse image.

But when Professor Smith and her students at Oregon Health and Science University later conducted a study of such greeting cards, they found more than the expected naughty nurse themes. There was also a focus on what an August 2003 Oregon Public Broadcasting piece on the study called the "sadistic shot giver." As Smith wrote in *Nursing Spectrum*:

> Patients may believe the greeting card image that [the nurse] will cause fear and anxiety, often threatening to inflict

pain while using devices such as syringes, thermometers, or whips....Disguised as humor, this disrespect and lack of understanding echoes back to the hard, commanding, uncaring image of Nurse Ratched in the movie *One Flew Over the Cuckoo's Nest*.[1]

Nurse Mildred Ratched is indeed the modern archetype of the nurse as battle-axe. Milos Forman's classic 1975 film adaptation of Ken Kesey's novel captures the anti-authoritarian spirit of the sixties counterculture. In the movie, Randle McMurphy is a charismatic roughneck who engineers a transfer from a work farm, where he has been serving a sentence for assault, to an Oregon state mental health facility he thinks will be easier. He joins a unit of men with psychiatric problems. Ratched dominates the unit, leading the patients in what at first seems like actual group therapy, and offering calm, rational explanations for an array of rules. But McMurphy gradually realizes that Ratched is a cunning sociopath who psychologically tortures those she is ostensibly helping, aided by the meek Nurse Pilbow. Ratched manipulates the young patient Billy through his fear of his mother, making Billy feel that his interest in sex is evil. Meanwhile, as absentee male physicians debate whether McMurphy is really ill, McMurphy works to undermine Ratched's authority. He leads the patients on forbidden adventures involving wine, women, and song, which plainly promote more healing than Ratched's joyless regime. As McMurphy's refusal to conform instills a sense of independence in the other patients, Ratched resorts to increasingly harsh measures to maintain control, with tragic results.

Nurse Ratched is a repressive soul killer. Even her name evokes words like "rat," "wretched," and "hatchet." And the film offers no positive counterexample or explanation for her behavior, such as burnout after years in a difficult care setting. Ratched could be a warning about the potential for abuse in the nursing profession, but she can't be separated from the film's views of women generally. They are either emasculating, anti-sex mother figures like Ratched, spineless mice like Pilbow, or easy, giggling facilitators like McMurphy's girlfriend, whose name is Candy. The movie indicts establishment power structures, suggesting that real men must reclaim their power and freedom from the oppressive modern state. But the film seems to place the blame mostly on Mom, who just won't let boys be boys. Of course it doesn't make much sense: women were not the main creators of those power structures. But no one said misogyny was rational. Evidently, Ratched is what happens when you *do* give women control. What kind of place is it where a *nurse* has more power than the *physicians*? A twisted, unnatural place, dominated by the Other.

The other important modern battle-axe was the Margaret "Hot Lips" Houlihan character in *M*A*S*H*. Robert Altman's innovative 1970 film about a U.S. Army surgical unit in the Korean War, based on the 1968 novel by Richard Hooker, mockingly dissects those involved in the military's effort there. The dark comedy is another anti-authoritarian classic with a viscerally misogynistic approach. The nurses who appear fall into the categories of naughty, handmaiden, and battle-axe. Major Houlihan, the unit's new chief nurse, is a martinet aghast at the unmilitary conduct she finds. She and the inept surgeon Frank Burns tattle to the military brass in Seoul, and they begin a cringe-inducing affair, though he is married. In response, the film's heroes, the cynical surgeons Hawkeye and Trapper, engineer a nasty invasion of privacy that humiliates Burns and Houlihan. Then our heroes implement a plan to determine Houlihan's true hair color that the film finds hilarious, but which has something in common with gang rape. After that, "Hot Lips" is more docile, Trapper praises her nursing, and she seems to earn some redemption by joining the surgeons' boyish fun.

In the popular television series that followed (1972–1983), the depiction of nursing was better. The show's nurses were still mostly assistants and easy romantic foils for the surgeons, who received virtually all the credit or blame for patient outcomes. But the series showed some actual nursing, and there was little doubt about Houlihan's authority over the nurses, her nursing skills, or her commitment to the patients. As the series went on, she grew increasingly sympathetic. Unlike Ratched, Houlihan made a clear positive difference for patients. However, especially in the early years, she was still a fairly pathetic martinet, grasping at power and petty discipline — and a man to fill the void in her career-dominated life, a struggle that was the subject of endless mockery. Houlihan was far more than a battle-axe, but the influential character still suggested that strong nurses are control freaks driven by half-repressed romantic urges.

Ratched and Houlihan set the standards for a certain type of fictional nursing image in later decades: the older female nurse as bitter crone and vindictive bureaucrat. In general, the battle-axe inverts both the maternal/angel image and the naughty image. She is yet another one-dimensional female extreme, a way to put women in their place if they are doing something you don't like. It may be that this image has resonated because of patients' feelings of vulnerability and anxiety at being at the mercy of female caregivers who would normally be in a subservient social position. The classic battle-axe has appeared in many Hollywood shows, often as the nasty enforcer of hospital rules that are presented as oppressive or trivial, even though some are actually vital to the patient's recovery.

A recent variation on the classic battle-axe is the malevolent hottie, a sexually aggressive younger "nurse" who poses a real or mock threat to patients or others. This fictional image, which we might call the "naughty-axe," has appeared in connection with horror films, ads, and video games. Perhaps foreshadowed by the naughty elements of "Hot Lips" Houlihan, the naughty-axe image seems to invert only the maternal stereotype. The naughty-axe does not oppose sex. But because the image does associate sexuality with danger, it is true to the underlying spirit of the classic battle-axe.

The troubled Oregon State Hospital where *Cuckoo's Nest* was filmed was scheduled to be torn down starting in late 2008. But nurse battle-axe imagery has persisted in the media. Why is that, since women have far more power in the workplace now? Do some nurses really act like vindictive bureaucrats? Of course some do, as in any profession. And that is especially unsurprising for an underpowered profession in the midst of a long staffing crisis. But battle-axe portrayals typically provide little balance or context to explain why some nurses might act that way. By contrast, there are many admiring portrayals of powerful female physicians. And those that do question their use of power often make clear how hard it still is for women to assert authority without being seen as "bitches."

So while modern society may be at least ambivalent about punishing women *generally* for exercising power, it remains acceptable to punish women for being powerful *nurses* — a practice even "feminists" engage in, as explained in chapter 6. Thus the nurse battle-axe is a safe outlet for feel-good regressive values. Enjoy that misogyny responsibly!

# TYRANTS, BUREAUCRATS, MONSTERS: HOLLYWOOD CELEBRATES NURSING AUTHORITY

Prime-time U.S. television rarely shows a positive nurse character with genuine authority. As we saw in chapters 3 and 4, several late 2005 *ER* episodes did feature the strong nurse manager Eve Peyton. Peyton was a strict micromanager, and one staff nurse suggested that she was a "bitch." But Peyton was also a clinical expert with a doctorate who seemed to care about patients. However, her departure marked a crude and implausible swerve into extreme battle-axe territory. In one December 2005 episode, Peyton got dumped by her boyfriend; decked an offensive patient and poured urine on him, with no physical provocation and no regret; was fired on Christmas Eve; and bid farewell to the ED staff with standard PhD-type phrases like "bite me," "screw yourselves," and "you all suck." Maybe this all seemed funny because many still consider nurses to be harmless "angels." But the episode is a bit less amusing when you consider that ED nurses are many times more likely to be the victims than the causes of workplace violence — something *ER* has rarely shown.

There has since been no significant *ER* nurse character to balance Peyton. Major nurse character Sam Taggart is expert, but she is not that senior and has no obvious authority. By comparison, *ER*'s depictions of harsh physician managers like Kerry Weaver and Robert Romano have been countered with many portraits of wise, humane ones, including women like Susan Lewis and Elizabeth Corday. On her way out, Peyton ranted that she "tried to elevate this stupid ER." But she was less a frustrated reformer than a nurse who had the temerity to push successfully against her *ER*-assigned role as physician subordinate. It's fine for women to be assertive in traditionally male professions like medicine. But aggressive nurses are too much of a threat to the natural order, and perhaps to the "feminist" doctrine that able women who choose health care careers must become physicians. So any assertive woman who chooses *nursing* must be a bitter, dangerous loon, frustrated in love — a battle-axe.

A memorable battle-axe also appeared in a January 2004 *ER*, when medical student Abby Lockhart does a rotation in the Neonatal Intensive Care Unit (NICU). This unit seems to be staffed mainly by physicians and medical students, rather than the nurses who staff it in real life. In this physician-intensive care unit, one of the two nurses who emerge from the wallpaper leaves the impression that veteran NICU nurses are martinets bent on terrorizing medical students. A NICU attending introduces nurse Virgie as a twenty-year veteran whose mission is to protect the babies from medical students. That is one thing NICU nurses do, but Virgie is hostile, rule-bound, and — contrary to the attending's introduction — apparently not concerned about the patients. Virgie refuses Lockhart's request that she give, without advance physician authorization, medication to a deteriorating patient to stop his full-body seizures. And when Lockhart (who is also a nurse) does it herself, Virgie whines that she will report Lockhart to the attending. Virgie makes no effort to intervene and stop the patient's seizures. Instead, she stands by focused on her charting as her patient teeters in crisis. Virgie also confronts Lockhart for having changed a diaper without weighing it, ruining her count of "ins and outs." Lockhart apologizes but notes that the diaper is now in the trash. Virgie snaps "Not good enough!" and insists that Lockhart find and weigh it. We get no explanation that ins and outs are critical measures of a newborn's health. The episode also includes Tom, a kind, cooperative nurse who defers to the students:

so much for protecting the babies. In any case, Virgie dominates the episode's vision of nursing. Not good enough!

*Grey's Anatomy* also tends to present senior nurses as vindictive bureaucrats who are always working against the young surgical heroes. In one November 2005 episode discussed in chapter 3, hotshot intern Cristina Yang steals an interesting case from the psychiatric ward. But cranky veteran nurse Debbie questions Cristina: "This room is supposed to be unoccupied. Whose patient is this?...Who transferred him? I don't have any paperwork, any transfer documents." Yang dismisses Debbie by noting that the physicians will let her know if a bedpan needs changing. The nurses retaliate by paging Yang to do disgusting scut work.

This absurd fantasy about workplace roles was likely a misguided effort to show nurses respect. But it does not suggest that disrespecting nurses is wrong or unsafe, merely that, as resident Miranda Bailey notes, it's "stupid" to antagonize the nurses. Debbie might have been shown humiliating Cristina by catching the intern's error and saving a patient's life. Or she might have simply explained what nursing really is. Instead, Debbie's revenge is that of a petty bureaucrat who really *is* all about bedpans. And Cristina has the last laugh. Recall Winston Churchill's response to a woman who told him he was drunk, one version of which is "I may be drunk, Miss, but in the morning I will be sober, and you will still be ugly." Cristina may have been a little drunk on ego and ambition, but in the morning of future episodes, she remains a pretty, esteemed surgeon. Debbie is still a disagreeable battle-axe who cleans up the mess.

Another notable battle-axe appeared on ABC's short-lived *MDs*, which aired in 2002. The drama tried to transplant the basic premise of *M*A*S*H* — two renegade surgeons thwarting a bad system to save lives — to a San Francisco hospital. Physicians provided all important care, but the show did not ignore nurses: one major character was "Nurse 'Doctor' Poole," who used her PhD — in management — to act as a heartless enforcer for the evil HMO that controlled the hospital. Poole was a Frankenstein made from the worst parts of Nurse Ratched and Margaret Houlihan, a bean-counting monster who relished denying patients needed care. Like Ratched, Poole used her training to control patients and undermine their health. Like Houlihan at her worst, Poole was obsessed with enforcing rules and frustrated by subversive surgeons who wouldn't conform. Poole, like Houlihan, even had a pathetic affair with a married cohort. Of course, some real nurses have been co-opted by the managed care system, but far more fight constantly to protect their patients from it. The crowning touch was Poole's "Doctor" label, which the show itself put in quotes. *MDs* mocked the very idea of a nurse with a doctorate and linked it with the perceived backwardness of managed care. What kind of system allows a *nurse* to pretend to be a doctor?

The nurse battle-axe has also graced non-health care shows. The September 2005 season premiere of CBS's *Cold Case* focused on an investigation involving a pro-life school nurse. Nurse Laura manipulated a high school couple into having their baby — lying to them about the effects of and legal requirements for abortion — and set in motion forces that destroyed their lives. Nurse Laura also had a record of arrests for assaulting clinic workers, and the show presented her as a moralizing hypocrite, herself having an affair with a married teacher (recall Houlihan and Poole).

Two months later an episode of NBC's *Law and Order* focused on the death of an abusive mother, who had been jailed for allegedly killing a man who reported her to child protective services. The mother's death was caused by a reaction to an IUD given to her by nurse Gloria, who was secretly sterilizing women she deemed

unworthy of having children. The show's district attorneys pros-
ecuted Gloria. Both shows included strong female law enforcement
characters.

These crime shows retooled Nurse Ratched for the modern
era. Neo-Ratched still embodies institutional oppression and sexual
intolerance: both nurses in these plots use their authority to deny
troubled women the right to make their own reproductive choices.
Unlike Ratched, the nurses are motivated by understandable goals.
But far beyond merely taking a principled stand against abortion
or child abuse, these nurses abdicate their ethical duties and actually hurt *women* — something Ratched did not do. Nursing seems
to be a backwater populated by zealots with no use for the lawful
avenues democracies offer to effect social change. Neo-Ratched is a
throwback who is actually dragging women back with her, doing a
job that enlightened women like our law enforcement heroes have
left behind. Only women who pursue traditionally male professions
are worthy of real power.

A March 2006 episode of HBO's *The Sopranos* finds gravely
wounded Mafia boss Tony Soprano in a coma and on a hospital ventilator. Tony's family and subordinates keep watch. Nurses appear
from time to time, but Tony's wife Carmela and daughter Meadow
take a far more active role in his care. They talk to the unconscious
Tony, they touch him, and Meadow even climbs into bed next to
him. Since none of the episode's nurses gets a name, we'll assign them
numbers. At one point Nurse 1 chastises Silvio, Tony's consigliere, as
he reads a newspaper at the nurse's station: "Sir, it's family only in the
unit." Silvio says he will be out of her hair in a minute. Nurse 1: "I
keep telling you people, I'm gonna have to call the hospital administrator." At another point, we see Nurse 1 working at the bedside,
emptying blood out of a drain. She exits, looking bitter and eyeing

Meadow and mob guy Paulie: "Only one person at a time, please." After she leaves, Meadow confirms, "She's a ball buster." At another point Carmela enters the comatose Tony's room as Nurse 2 is adjusting his tubes. Nurse 2 snaps, "Don't get in bed with him again, you dislodged his drains." Carmela: "That was my daughter, and I can't help but think that physical affection means something." Nurse 2 shakes her head as if Carmela is deranged. Later, after Tony has been out of the coma for some time, Carmela enters his room to find him sitting in a chair. She asks Nurse 3, "You've got him up?" Nurse 3: "I know how it looks, but he should be upright as much as possible." Nurse 3 does not explain why. Instead, she checks something and leaves quickly.

Nurse 3 is not too bad, but on the whole, the episode portrays ICU nurses as nasty, rule-bound bureaucrats who actually impede psychosocial care. There is no context to explain why that might be, no indication of poor workplace conditions, no indication even that the nurses find that dealing with a group of mass murderers makes them a little edgy. And viewers are unlikely to see the importance of any of the rules the nurses enforce. No one explains. Of course, pulling out drains could result in serious complications, but nurses should and do still help families find ways to provide physical affection to patients. In fact, however realistic it is, this episode suggests that Tony is brought back from the edge of death by awareness of his loved ones' presence. In effect, the message is that nurses could learn something about psychosocial care and family presence from the Mafia family. Maybe Carmela and Meadow could put together some clinical training for them!

As discussed in chapter 5, recent horror films have used naughty-axe imagery, which in one neat package provides the fear and sexuality that often drive those films. For the Halloween 2006 release *Saw*

*III*, Lion's Gate and Twisted Pictures promoted a related blood drive with posters featuring sexy/scary "naughty nurse" imagery. Nurses also figured in the 2006 horror film *Silent Hill* and the Konami video games on which the film was based. These nurses were at times presented sexually, but they were also deformed monsters who manifested human fears — not a bad definition of a battle-axe. And in the 2006 *Candy Stripers,* a hospital full of sexy, horny "candy striper nurses" are bent on spreading a horrific alien virus with which they had been infected. Characters like these differ greatly from the classic battle-axe, but they achieve a similar effect: to link nurses who actually have power with malevolence.

## HOVERING LIKE GHOULS: BATTLE-AXES IN OTHER MEDIA

The battle-axe appears in a variety of recent media, in both her classic and naughty-axe forms. In 2005 the Kentucky company Diversified Designs ran an ad for its CompuCaddy computer stands in magazines such as *Health Data Management*. In the ad, a furious "nurse" points her finger and bares her teeth. She wears a severe, traditional white uniform, and her name tag reads "HELEN WHEELS, R.N." The caption: "The morning shift would like a word with you!" Helen is mad because her computer stand battery is dead: the idea is that CompuCaddy would help prevent this crisis because its batteries last longer. Of course, any nurse in Helen's situation might be displeased, but the character's "hell on wheels" name and general presentation suggest that she is an ogre to be avoided under any circumstances.

But that's nothing. In T. Coraghessan Boyle's short story "Chicxulub," nurses are cold martinets who represent the mindless brutality of the universe. No, really. The story appeared in *The New Yorker* in March 2004 and in Boyle's 2005 collection *Tooth and Claw*. It compares the potential loss of a couple's beloved teenage daughter to the ever-present possibility that a big rock will strike the Earth and end civilization. The father/narrator describes the night he and his wife are called to the hospital following a serious car accident. Arriving at what appears to be the Emergency Department, the couple approaches the "admittance desk." The young "Filipina" nurse there greets the distraught couple by demanding, "Name?" She has "opaque eyes and the bone structure of a cadaver; every day she sees death and it blinds her. She doesn't see us." Retrieving information from her computer with her "fleshless fingers," the nurse refuses to tell them anything more than that their daughter is still in surgery. The father wonders why he "despise[s] this nurse more than any human being [he's] ever encountered" — this woman "with her hair pulled back in a bun and a white cap like a party favor perched atop it, *who is just doing her job*?" Why does he want to "reach across the counter that separates us and awaken her to a swift, sure knowledge of hate and fear and pain? Why?"

The desperate couple proceeds to surgery, "and here is another nurse, grimmer, older, with lines like the strings of a tobacco pouch pulled tight around her lips." The couple asks if their daughter will be all right. "'I don't have that information,' the nurse says, and her voice is neutral, robotic even. This is not her daughter." The father can't handle this "maddening clinical neutrality" and he explodes, suggesting that it's the nurse's job to know what's going on after the couple has been dragged in and told their daughter has been hurt. The nurse "drills" the father with a look. She steps away from her desk, revealing herself to be "short," "dumpy," and "almost a dwarf." She leads the couple to a room, saying, "Wait here.... The doctor will be in in a minute." Then she disappears, leaving them alone there for "a good hour or more." Won't someone rescue this poor couple from the clutches of modern nursing? Someone will, as a young surgeon finally appears and offers the only decent words the parents have heard at this hospital. Then he leads them through what sounds like an ICU, where patients are surrounded by machines with "nurses hovering over them like ghouls."

Of course, nurses who work in stressful conditions can behave badly, but the extreme battle-axe vision that this sympathetic narrator presents is hard to miss, and Boyle gives us no real reason to question it. Yes, the father is upset. But consider the dramatic ascent from the ugly, hateful nurses to the sensitive physician who will actually give them information and who has apparently been trying to save the couple's daughter all by himself. The nurses guard their computers or hover like "ghouls," protecting themselves by brutalizing distraught family members. They are inhuman bookkeepers of death.

The naughty-axe image also figures in various pop culture products. In particular, the hottie as "sadistic shot giver" wielding an enormous phallic syringe seems to be a cool way for pop musicians to move product. As we explained in chapter 5, a 2004 Skechers ad campaign featured naughty nurse Christina Aguilera brandishing an enormous syringe connected to a big needle, and the band blink-182 used a porn star as a naughty nurse flaunting another huge syringe in the artwork of a 1999 album.

But naughty-axes don't just look threatening, they also kick ass. Two popular recent wrestling video games have featured sexy "nurse" images. In Yuke's WWE SmackDown! vs. Raw 2006, gamers competing in barely dressed female "nurse" and other modes can slap, kick, and grapple, toss each other on a bouncy bed, rip each other's clothes off, and spank each other. Yeah, baby.

Konami's Rumble Roses games, released in 2004 and 2006, featured an evil naughty nurse character named Anesthesia. She had devastating moves and was also, needless to say, using the body parts of her victims to create a malevolent cyborg to help her rule the world. Of course, as we've noted, real nurses are the health workers most likely to be the victims of workplace violence.

At the risk of being labeled battle-axes, we have to say that the continuing appearance of battle-axe imagery suggests that, for many, nursing remains caught in an ugly cultural time warp. Female nurses with any power must be threatening, frustrated, and/or disagreeable. Yes, the media tells us, some women today can handle real authority — women with brains and education. But a good nurse's role is submission.

# CHAPTER 9

# Advanced Practice Nurses: Skilled Professionals or Cut-Rate "Physician Extenders"?

I N 2002 A GROUP OF RESIDENT physicians was conducting rounds at Johns Hopkins, perhaps the most well-regarded hospital in the United States. The senior resident pointed out to the medical interns a group of nurse practitioners (NPs) doing their patient rounds. The resident suggested, with heavy irony, that if the interns *really* wanted to learn what was going on, they should join the NPs! The idea was that the NPs were inconsequential pretenders to the physician throne.

In late 2005 Mattel, the world's leading toy maker, released a small collectible duck doll called the Nurse Quacktitioner. Dressed in a white lab coat and a white cap with a red heart on it, the doll sold at Target, Wal-Mart, and other major toy retailers. Whatever Mattel's intent, the name suggested that NPs are "quacks," untrained persons who pretend to be physicians. Mattel said it had no idea that this doll would be taken as an attack on NPs, whose main professional stereotype has been that they are, uh, untrained persons who pretend to be physicians. The company explained that the name included the word "quack" because ducks quack, a point that had *completely* eluded the more than two thousand nurses who objected to the doll. Mattel refused to remove the doll before the end of its planned run, even after the Center for Nursing Advocacy convinced Wal-Mart to sell the dolls back to Mattel.

Meanwhile, physicians in the UK learned of the controversy, and many sent letters of support — to Mattel, urging the company to keep selling the doll because it *would* foster contempt for NPs. The physicians argued that NPs are indeed unqualified practitioners (well, quacks) used to cut costs at the expense of quality care.

In fact, a large body of research shows that the care of NPs and other advanced practice registered nurses (APRNs) is at least as effective as that of physicians. In the 1960s nurses began training as advanced practitioners in primary care and other fields that included work traditionally done by physicians. Advanced practice nursing evolved mainly to provide care to disadvantaged persons who were not receiving physician care. Advanced practice nurses, most with at least a master's degree, now provide care in many specialties. They practice mainly in the United States but increasingly in other nations as well. APRNs are especially likely to provide care to underserved urban and rural populations. Like other nurses, APRNs employ a holistic care model that emphasizes prevention, health maintenance, and overall quality of life. APRNs are adept at identifying subtle problems and managing serious chronic conditions.

In the United States there were about 240,000 advanced practice nurses in 2004. More than 140,000 are NPs, specializing in many fields. More than 32,000 certified registered nurse anesthetists (CRNAs) provide most of the anesthesia given in the United States.

More than 14,000 certified nurse midwives (CNMs) provide ob/gyn care and deliver babies using a natural care model, one many other developed nations use to achieve better patient outcomes at lower cost. And more than 70,000 graduate-prepared clinical nurse specialists (CNSs) provide clinical leadership to direct care nurses.[1]

In the new millennium, direct care nurses suffered the effects of the global shortage, and nurse midwives struggled to cope with increasing practice costs. CNSs had grown in number and improved care greatly through the early 1990s, but hospitals eliminated many CNS positions in the managed care era, undermining clinical leadership in nursing. Still, the practice of NPs and CRNAs continued to expand. NP-staffed health clinics based in retail stores — like those selling the Nurse Quacktitioner — grew quickly. Nursing leaders now plan to establish the existing four-year doctorate of nursing practice (DNP) degree as the standard for all new APRNs by 2015. These last two developments sparked fierce resistance from some physician groups. However, cost-effective NP-directed care offers not only a way to enhance access to care for underserved populations, but also an advanced hybrid practice model that could change the future of health care for everyone.

Media portrayals of APRNs have been mixed. Hollywood has offered a few well-meaning television portrayals that have, at their best, suggested that NPs are moderately skilled assistants to physicians. At their worst (as in *Private Practice*), they have expressed overt contempt. Some news stories have conveyed a good sense of APRN practice, for instance in reporting on physician efforts to limit APRN practice and on the growth of the DNP degree. But APRNs continue to be ignored as general health experts, and the media's relentless suggestions that practitioner care is provided only by "doctors" continue unabated in news pieces and advertising. Doubt it? Just "ask your doctor"! Some press accounts have wrongly suggested that APRNs are capable only of treating minor problems. Very often, the media allows physicians to express uninformed criticism without consulting APRNs or the relevant research.

However, some media creators, including physicians, are receptive to the idea that APRNs make valuable contributions to modern health care. In 2002 the U.S. Department of Health and Human Services (HHS) launched an annual campaign to increase visits to primary care providers. It was called Take a Loved One to the Doctor Day. The Center for Nursing Advocacy led nurses in trying to persuade HHS to change the name to one that would not exclude the APRNs who provide vital primary care to the very minority populations the campaign targets. In July 2005 HHS — with the leadership of Assistant Secretary for Minority Health Garth Graham, MD, MPH — actually changed the name, to Take a Loved One for a Checkup Day. HHS gave its campaign partners discretion to use the old name, and popular ABC Radio host Tom Joyner and some others insisted on doing so. But many others embraced the new name. Next up: Improve a Loved One's Understanding of APRNs Day!

## WHO ARE APRNs AND HOW GOOD IS THEIR CARE?

APRNs are skilled health professionals who provide advanced holistic care, including diagnosis and treatment traditionally done by physicians, in a great variety of settings. These range from major teaching hospitals to small clinics, and from the military to public health services.

Because APRNs take a holistic approach, they are especially skilled at cost-effective preventative care, the management of chronic disease, coordinating care among different providers, and long-term health maintenance. Many APRNs focus on underserved poor communities where physicians choose not to practice, so APRNs are a vital health resource for millions who would otherwise receive little or no health care. APRNs' work has become even more critical as fewer physicians choose to pursue less lucrative primary care practices. On the other hand, some nursing advocates have argued that the growth in APRN practice has drawn nurses away from the bedside and from teaching positions, exacerbating the nursing shortage. In an era in which severe short-staffing has made bedside practice difficult, these are understandable concerns.

The first NP program (in pediatrics) was developed by public health nurse Loretta Ford, EdD, and pediatrician Henry Silver, MD, at the University of Colorado in 1965. Today NP specialties include family practice, intensive care, emergency care, oncology, cardiology, mental health, and surgery, among many others. As described by the American Academy of Nurse Practitioners,

> NPs are advanced practice nurses who provide high-quality health care services similar to those of a doctor. NPs diagnose and treat a wide range of health problems. They have a unique approach and stress both care and cure. Besides clinical care, NPs focus on health promotion, disease prevention, health education and counseling. They help patients make wise health and lifestyle choices.[2]

Nurse anesthetists provide highly skilled, cost-effective anesthesia services. Nurse midwives provide ob/gyn and prenatal care, and deliver babies under a care model that treats the birth process as a natural one, rather than an illness. And clinical nurse specialists are APRNs who provide vital clinical leadership to direct care nurses and provide direct care in some community settings. They practice in a variety of specialties, including pediatrics, geriatrics, emergency care, critical care, and psychiatric care. The U.S. National Association of Clinical Nurse Specialists explains:

> In addition to providing direct patient care, Clinical Nurse Specialists influence care outcomes by providing expert consultation for nursing staffs and by implementing improvements in health care delivery systems. Clinical Nurse Specialist practice integrates nursing practice, which focuses on assisting patients in the prevention or resolution of illness, with medical diagnosis and treatment of disease, injury and disability.[3]

In the United States APRNs are licensed by each state, bound by legal and ethical duties, and subject to malpractice actions. Their legal rights to practice without collaborating with physicians vary by state. APRNs are eligible for Medicare and Medicaid reimbursement, and they can prescribe most medications. In some states, APRNs run successful independent health practices, though the extent of their rights to prescribe medication and to receive insurance reimbursement has been hotly disputed.

Some people regard physician training as superior to that of APRNs. Physician training in the United States includes a four-year undergraduate degree with some rigorous science courses and a demanding four-year graduate medical degree, in addition to several years of training in residency programs. On the other hand, APRNs have a four-year bachelor's degree in nursing science, two or more years of intense graduate education in nursing science, and the informal training in the first years of APRN practice that any serious professional receives. In most cases, they also have years of highly relevant experience practicing as RNs before their graduate educa-tion. Some APRNs have doctorates.[4] APRNs are trained to provide care that addresses all facets of human well-being.

Nevertheless, some physician groups have questioned the safety of APRN care and fought to restrict the scope of APRN practice, claiming that APRNs require physician "supervision," as some state laws still provide. Many physicians, and even some APRNs, refer to APRNs as "physician extenders" or "mid-level providers." These con-temptuous terms suggest that APRNs are the extremities of physi-cians, perhaps helping them reach things on a high shelf, and also that only physicians are "high-level" (presumably RNs are "low-level"). Of course, the term "advanced practice" nurse itself may suggest that RNs are not advanced, and this term could probably be improved.

We are aware of no scientific basis for physicians' safety claims about APRNs. In fact, a vast body of research indicates that the care of APRNs is at least as good as that of physicians.[5] For example, as the American Academy of Nurse Anesthetists has noted, "No studies to date that have addressed anesthesia care outcomes have found that there is a significant difference in patient outcomes based on whether the anesthesia provider is a [certified nurse anesthetist] or [a physician] anesthesiologist."[6] That finding should not be surprising in view of APRNs' rigorous training and patient-focused practice model.

Some studies have found differences, but overall these have tended to suggest that if any practitioners' care is better, it is that of APRNs. For instance, in June 2003 the *American Journal of Public Health* published a study of low-risk obstetric patients funded by the U.S. Agency for Health Care Research and Quality. The study compared two groups of patients. Group 1 received birth center care from a team in which 95 percent of care was delivered by certified nurse midwives and 5 percent of care came from OB physicians. Patients in Group 2 received care only from physicians. The two groups had comparable rates of morbidity, preterm birth, and low birth weight. But in other respects, the 95 percent nurse midwife team care resulted in better outcomes and a lower cost, as patients spent less time as inpatients and had fewer C-sections, episiotomies, inductions, and vacuum- or forceps-assisted vaginal births.[7]

In April 2002, Horrocks, Anderson, & Salisbury published a meta-analysis of thirty-four clinical studies in the *British Medical Journal* indicating that patients were more satisfied with their care if it was delivered by an NP than if by a physician. NPs read X-rays equally well, identified more physical abnormalities, communicated better, and taught patients how to provide self-care better. NPs also spent more time with patients than did physicians (14.9 versus 11.2 minutes).[8]

In January 2000 researchers from the Columbia University School of Nursing published a randomized clinical study of 1,316 patients in the *Journal of the American Medical Association* comparing nurse practitioners and physicians. Patients answered a satisfaction questionnaire after their initial appointment and were examined six months and one year later. At six months, physicians received a higher satisfaction rating (4.2 versus 4.1 on a 5.0 scale). However, there were no differences in the use of health care resources, and the only difference in outcomes was that the nurse practitioner patients who suffered from high blood pressure had significantly lower diastolic blood pressures than comparable physician patients did.[9]

And in November 1995 Brown and Grimes from the University of Texas at Austin School of Nursing published a meta-analysis of thirty-three studies in the journal *Nursing Research*. The analysis compared the outcomes of primary care patients of NPs and certified nurse midwives (CNMs) with those of physicians. Patients of NPs had significantly greater adherence with treatment recommendations than patients of physicians. Patients of NPs also had higher satisfaction and better resolution of pathological conditions than patients of physicians. CNMs used less technology and analgesia during labor and delivery, and the two groups of providers delivered babies with similar outcomes.[10]

Nursing leaders plan to make the doctorate of nursing practice (DNP) degree the standard APRN degree by 2015, as noted above. The DNP degree includes four years of graduate education, plus a one-year residency, after the bachelor's degree. In addition to providing fodder for hilarious "Dr. Nurse" wordplay, the idea appears to be to expand the knowledge base of APRNs and to promote greater parity with primary care physicians. Some nurses have expressed concerns that the move could effectively require current APRNs to obtain more graduate education, that it implies current APRN abilities are inadequate, and that it could lead to the "medicalization" of APRN practice.

Predictably, the plan has also encountered strong resistance from the physician groups that have tried to limit APRN practice. They argue that further "blurring the lines" between the professions will endanger patient health. In June 2008 the American Medical Association's House of Delegates passed one resolution stating that DNPs should be supervised by physicians, and another stating that the National Board of Medical Examiners should not, as planned, offer a certifying exam for DNPs. But the delegates rejected a proposed resolution seeking to limit the use of the terms "doctor" and "residency" in clinical settings to physicians, dentists, and podiatrists. That proposal would have prevented not just nurses but also psychologists, social workers, and others from describing their own qualifications. Maybe the problem was that the proposal did not go far enough. To really protect the physician brand, we suggest barring the very issuance of doctorates in any field but medicine. Nurses aren't the only ones who need to learn their place!

"Doctor" jokes aside, we believe that APRNs have developed a hybrid care model with the potential to revolutionize advanced practitioner care. Are they the ones to help liberate the public from the current health care morass?

## "MIDWIFS" AND MINOR AILMENTS: APRNs IN HOLLYWOOD

Hollywood has taken some notice of APRNs, particularly NPs and nurse midwives. Television shows have presented some ostensibly positive visions of APRNs, but they have also suggested that APRNs treat only simple conditions in an environment rightly controlled by physicians. No major television product has really conveyed the nature or value of the APRN practice model. Probably the most notable recent portrayals have been the nurse midwifery characters on *Strong Medicine* (2000–2006) and on *Private Practice* (launched in 2007), which has repeatedly mocked nurse midwifery. And recent films have generally ignored APRNs, though there have been helpful minor depictions in Mike Nichols's 2003 *Angels in America* and Abby Epstein's 2008 documentary *The Business of Being Born*.

*Strong Medicine*'s nurse midwife character Peter Riggs has probably been serial television's best portrayal of an APRN. He did not figure heavily in most episodes, and he did not spend much time actually delivering babies or seeing outpatients, as a real nurse midwife would. But he did seem to operate with some autonomy, treating patients in a clinic run by primary care physician Luisa Delgado. One

September 2005 episode had Riggs establishing and skillfully running a "baby boot camp" for gangbanging boyfriends of his patients who were not meeting their fathering responsibilities. Riggs clearly took a holistic approach to care, which the show both honored and poked fun at. Riggs reported to Delgado and the show's other physicians, and he generally deferred to them in clinical matters, with minor exceptions. In one episode, Riggs did confront a powerful ob-gyn who had performed an unnecessary C-section, resulting in a hysterectomy, and Delgado had to save Riggs's job, as discussed in chapter 6. In the September 2005 episode mentioned above, Riggs briefly argued with a major surgeon character about which of them had delivered more babies and so would be more qualified to deliver Delgado's. And in the February 2006 series finale, Riggs resisted pressure from his girlfriend, a physician resident, to go to medical school. Riggs said he preferred to be a nurse, though he gave only the vague reason that medicine would not make him "happier." Viewers got no sense that he regarded advanced practice nursing to be as valuable as medicine generally.

Peter Riggs had his moments, but as we've seen, the Dell Parker character on *Private Practice* is an APRN disaster. A receptionist with a "nursing degree" who is studying to be a midwife, Dell seems to know little about health care. Early episodes mocked midwifery, as superstar ob-gyn Addison Montgomery uttered the word "midwif" as if she had never heard of such an outlandish pursuit. In the September 2007 series premiere, Dell asked her if he could help with a delivery for "field experience for my midwife training" — as if his clinical training consisted of whatever ad hoc assistance he could offer clinic physicians, rather than the midwife-directed graduate degree training he would get in real life. Addison repeatedly rejected his help. Dell eventually lost it:

*Dell:* You don't take me seriously.... You think I'm some dumb surfer boy, you think I'm eye candy. You have no respect for me or my midwifery skills.

*Addison (struggling not to laugh):* I have total respect for you and your... mid*wife*ry skills? Is that even a word — mid*wife*ry?

*Dell (petulantly):* It's a word. (Pause.) It's definitely a word!

He walks off, impotent. Addison sighs. Of course the show is poking fun at the elite surgeon surrounded by Southland nuts, but it's also laughing at Dell's midwifery. Even accounting for Addison's arrogance, which the show celebrates by pretending to condemn, it's unlikely that an OB would really be unfamiliar with the word *midwifery*. But Addison doesn't know about it, we assume, because it's irrelevant to serious maternal-child health care. And receptionist Dell is not likely to cite the studies showing that nurse midwives' care is at least as effective as that provided by OBs like Addison.

On other major recent hospital shows, APRNs are conspicuously absent. Even the most realistic, NBC's *ER*, has never had a major APRN character. The show did include a brief appearance by an APRN in the Carol Hathaway era of the 1990s, and the nurse character Sam Taggart did start a nurse anesthetist program in fall 2008. But as discussed in chapters 3 and 6, *ER* has often suggested that nurses achieve by going to medical school, when in reality they are one hundred times more likely to attend graduate nursing school.[11]

Both *House* and *Scrubs* have had nurse characters confront the idea of becoming NPs, though both sent damaging messages about NP education. A February 2007 *House* episode included nurse Wendy, the girlfriend of House's underling physician Foreman. Foreman cleverly breaks up with Wendy by telling her that he'll make "a few calls" and get her into an elite hospital-based NP program in a distant city. This plotline will likely suggest to most viewers that the most prestigious NP preparation is non-degree training to which entry can be had at the whim of physicians, rather than NP-directed graduate degree programs at major universities with rigorous admissions requirements.

The treatment of NP education on *Scrubs* was oddly similar. In a November 2002 episode, surgeon Turk signs up his future wife, nurse Carla Espinosa, for an NP program as a surprise gift. Unlike Foreman, Turk is trying to do something nice, and the episode makes clear that Carla is well qualified for the program: attending physician Perry Cox says so! But Carla chooses not to pursue it so she can spend more time with Turk. That's fair enough, but no one on the show argues that perhaps her nursing career is as important as Turk's physician career. And the subtler messages about NPs are similar to those in the *House* episode. Like Foreman, physician Turk apparently has the power to simply enroll Carla in the NP training, as if it was a beginner's class in ballroom dancing at the local community center. In both episodes, the nurses' boyfriends seem to assume that any nurse would leap at the chance to leave the bedside to pursue NP training. The nurse characters do not leap, for their own reasons, but neither defends bedside nursing either.

In late 2004 CBS aired *dr. vegas*, a flashy, short-lived drama about a Las Vegas casino physician named Billy Grant. Grant's casino clinic sidekick was NP Alice Doherty. Doherty was a skilled assistant to Grant with no real autonomy. She did show some health knowledge and a willingness to push Grant for more holistic care. At one point she argued successfully for alcoholic rehabilitation for an abusive patient when Grant wanted to treat the man's minor wounds and cut him loose. However, Doherty was also a little too romantically available.

It wasn't just that she had a big crush on Grant, eventually seducing him. The show also reinforced the old stereotype that romance with nurses is part of patients' therapy. An emaciated dying patient told Doherty that a date with her would help him cross an item off his to-do-before-dying list. And they actually had a dinner date, followed by innuendo from Grant about how far Doherty went.

The final episode of *dr. vegas* delivered a remarkably direct attack on NP competence and autonomy. Doherty, struggling to handle her unrequited love for Grant, got drunk with the ne'er-do-well son of the casino manager's old friend. Then, when this son injured himself on the casino dance floor, Doherty brought him back to the clinic and forged Grant's signature on an OxyContin prescription. Meanwhile, her date stole the prescription pad, resulting in keen interest from the police, especially when a hotel guest later OD'd and almost died. Grant saved the day by telling the police that he had authorized Doherty to write the prescription. The plotline presented a vision of the irresponsible NP, that flighty female who can't handle her romance or her liquor, and needless to say can't be trusted with the awful power of the prescription pad.

In September 2004, the syndicated television quiz show *Jeopardy!* included a clue about NPs. On the show, contestants receive the answer to a question, and they must provide the correct question to win points. In this episode, there was an "answer" stating, "Minor ailments can be treated by NPs (nurse practitioners) & PAs (these)." The contestant responded "correctly" by saying, "What are physician's assistants?" This answer wrongly suggested that major ailments like cardiac disease, cancer, and diabetes are beyond NPs. Nurses contacted the show with their concerns, and in June 2005 an episode featured this clue: "The Golden Lamp Awards are bestowed for the best portrayals of these health professionals in the media."

The Center for Nursing Advocacy gives these awards annually to recognize good (and bad) portrayals of nursing. Although we might have preferred a clue that communicated more of the substance of nursing, the way the clue played out illustrated the very attitudes that lead to poor understanding of NPs and nurses generally. Upon the reading of the clue, one of the three contestants — a medical student — quickly, almost gleefully, responded, "What are doctors?"

Hollywood films have generally taken little notice of APRNs. However, Mike Nichols's 2003 HBO adaptation of Tony Kushner's *Angels in America*, discussed in previous chapters, does include the NP Emily, a minor character who directs the major character Prior's AIDS care. No physician is shown treating Prior. Emily expertly assesses his condition, monitors his treatment, and helps him confront his fears. Emily does not share Prior's cultural knowledge — she has not heard of the Bayeux Tapestry — but her constancy and positivity make Prior's friend Louis look painfully inadequate.

And Abby Epstein's 2008 documentary *The Business of Being Born* offers a compelling argument that the United States return to an empowering midwifery-driven home birth model. The film presents U.S. obstetric care as a dysfunctional business that has consigned midwives to the periphery so that physicians who don't understand natural birth can perform dangerous, unnecessary interventions. Meanwhile, the film contends, the rest of the developed world achieves better outcomes for less money using midwives for most births. The film is not the portrayal of *nursing* care that it might have been. It largely ignores the work of nurse midwives in hospitals, and it never explains how nurse midwives differ from other midwives. However, the film does include a powerful portrait of New York City nurse midwife Cara Muhlhahn. Muhlhahn comes off as a birth expert as she visits patients and delivers babies. And she is articulate and passionate in explaining her role as "guardian of safety" and "witness to [the mother's] process."

# THE DOCTORATE OF SPLINTER DIAGNOSIS: APRNs IN THE NEWS MEDIA

The news media's treatment of APRNs has been mixed. They have received some good coverage as a new wave in health care, even as an alternative to the physician practitioner model. Marveling at APRN autonomy, patient satisfaction, and even skill, positive articles have focused particularly on the work of NPs and nurse midwives. Nurse anesthetists do not appear to have received as much fair coverage, and clinical nurse specialists appear to receive little coverage of any kind.

But the vast majority of media items about the work of advanced health practitioners simply ignore APRNs, casually discussing the work of "doctors" even when APRNs play a critical role in the care at issue. Prominent advertising for drugs typically advises the audience to "ask your doctor" about the advertised product. And many news items about APRN care show contempt for it, often relying solely on uninformed criticism from physicians rather than the relevant scientific research. If a physician says it, it must be true! These physician objections seem to have intensified as APRNs work increasingly in middle-class care settings in which physicians themselves are more likely to have an economic interest.

## Fair Reporting on APRNs

Some recent reports have described the growing role of NPs in primary care, with a particular focus on the NPs' expansion beyond care for the underserved communities they have traditionally served. The pieces often link this expansion to the decline in the number of primary care physicians. Andrew Blackman wrote an extraordinarily good October 2004 *Wall Street Journal* article of this type: "Is There a Doctor in the House? Perhaps Not, as Nurse Practitioners Take On Many of the Roles Long Played by Physicians." Blackman reports that nurse-run primary care practices "may be critical to the future of health care in the U.S." The story suggests that NPs' holistic, thorough, preventative approach may be uniquely suited to an aging population with long-term illnesses. In particular, the piece explains how the nurses' focus on patients' environments, psychological factors, and practical issues leads to solutions to long-term problems. Blackman discusses hurdles that NPs have yet to overcome, including legislative limits on their autonomy and the pay disparity with physicians doing comparable work. He acknowledges that "for many people the image of a nurse is still that of a junior partner to the all-knowing physician." Noting the concerns of some patients that NPs might miss a diagnosis, the article concludes that "studies have shown that when it comes to patient outcomes, nurse practitioners are just as good as doctors."

At the core of Blackman's piece is its description of the Columbia Advanced Practice Nurse Associates (Capna), a pioneering NP-run practice founded in 1994 by the Columbia University School of Nursing. Capna was the first nurse-run clinic in the United States to win full privileges to admit patients to hospitals, and the first to gain insurance compensation at the same rate as physicians. One Capna patient, a public relations professor, praises the comprehensive, unhurried approach of the NPs. She faults the physicians she saw before finding Capna, who she says had "no bedside manner" and just wanted to get patients out of the office quickly. Another patient compares NP-physician collaboration to his own experience as a business school graduate in partnership with a lawyer, a collaboration of two professions that approach issues in different ways but work well together. This patient suggests that perhaps "the future of health care is to find a way to combine the different skills of each one." However, the piece makes clear that NPs today are not just filling gaps but winning over patients who could easily be seeing physicians instead. Columbia nursing dean and Capna founder Mary Mundinger emphasizes that she chose an exclusive Madison Avenue address for one Capna office precisely so the NPs could compete directly with physicians.

Other reports emphasize APRNs' focus on underserved populations. In April 2004, the *Atlanta Journal-Constitution* ran a very good article by Patricia Guthrie about local NP Dorothy Gallaway. Gallaway's clinic provided low-income families with vital primary care and preventative health services, such as vaccinations, family planning, STD diagnosis, and treatment of high blood pressure and asthma. Gallaway said the clinic was also "seeing more insured patients because they like nurse practitioners."

And in November 2003, in discussing the growing role of primary care centers run by NPs, *Philadelphia Daily News* columnist Ronnie Polaneczky stressed that the centers could be vital in a state with a reported shortage of primary care physicians. She described a clinic in a public housing development that was run by NPs who "do everything primary-care physicians do." Polaneczky explained that there were more than a hundred such nurse-managed centers serving more than 1 million patients in thirty states. The article noted that research shows that, compared to patients in more traditional care settings, the nursing center patients saw their practitioners more often but used emergency departments 15 percent less and enjoyed shorter hospital maternity stays, lower prescription costs, and more effective preventative child health programs. Polaneczky asked whether "this excellent model of health-care delivery [could] be adapted for the mainstream."

Nurse midwives have received some attention, perhaps because of recent interest in different approaches to birthing. In July 2008, the *Post and Courier* (Charleston, SC) ran Jill Coley's report on the Charleston Birth Place as a new alternative for mothers who want a natural birth but also access to emergency care if needed. The Birth Place's owner, nurse midwife and family NP Lesley Rathbun, notes that a "culture of fear" has developed around birth in the United States, with women in labor "screaming" in the popular media. And in January 2006 Rhode Island's *Providence Journal* ran a glowing profile of nurse midwife Mary Breckinridge by Stanley M. Aronson, MD, dean of medicine emeritus at Brown University. "Kentucky's Intrepid Nurses on Horseback" discusses key elements of Breckinridge's globally influential work in founding and leading the Frontier Nursing Service, which has provided care to poor mothers and children in rural areas since 1925. The piece notes that today fourth-year Brown medical students "may spend up to three months in rural service supervised by these indomitable nurse midwives."

There has been some good coverage of threats to the midwives' practice. In a powerful May 2007 cover story in the *Washington Post Magazine*, Ly Phuong described the struggle of midwifery pioneer Ruth Lubic to keep birth centers for low-income urban women open, despite rising malpractice rates during the U.S. obstetric "liability crisis." Lubic "defied doctors to transform the way American women give birth." Over the past several decades, despite fierce resistance, Lubic established nurse midwife–staffed birthing centers in New York City and Washington, DC. The centers offered women an empowering and often safer alternative to the interventionist medical birth model. And in March 2004 the *New York Times* ran a fairly balanced article by Richard Pérez-Peña about the difficulties nurse midwives face, mainly far higher malpractice premiums and hospital- and insurance-imposed limits on their practices. Hospitals pointed to the insurance costs and an increase in high-risk pregnancies, but midwives suggested that factors included defensive care, hospital cost cutting, and physician fear of competition.

Other items have highlighted disputes over the scope of NP prac- tice. The *Savannah Morning News* posted Don Lowery's July 2005 story about a local primary care physician serving an eight-month sentence in federal prison, apparently in part for signing blank Schedule II substance prescription refills for NP colleagues to use. Such NP prescription was then unlawful in Georgia, though in no other U.S. state. The physician reportedly wrote the prescriptions so that he and the NPs with whom he practiced at a rural clinic could handle their huge patient load. The following year Georgia NPs finally gained statutory prescription authority. In March 2007 the *Atlanta Journal-Constitution* ran an editorial by Mike King force- fully opposing a proposal to roll back that prescription authority.

Some news outlets have reported on the plan to make the DNP the standard APRN degree by 2015. In April 2008 the *Wall Street Journal* ran Laura Landro's generally fair article "Making Room for 'Dr. Nurse.'" The piece presents the DNP degree, pioneered at Columbia University, as a "possible solution" to the decline in U.S. primary care physicians. Landro acknowledges that some current APRNs feel that they do not need the doctorate. She also explains that while some fear the DNP standard will lure nurses away from the bedside, others think it may create more nurse educators. The article describes the care patient Judith Gleason receives at Capna, whose DNPs she praises for their preventative care and keen diag- nostic skills. Gleason says of her DNP, "Edwidge is my primary-care provider now." The article falls short, however, when it says that NPs "fear the doctoral programs might be raising the bar too high for their profession," a distortion that implies either that nurses think they can't handle doctoral training or that nursing is not important enough to warrant it.

## The News Media Often Ignores or Disrespects APRNs

APRNs are rarely mentioned or consulted in health items that are not specifically about them. A constant assumption in the news media's treatment of health issues is that only "doctors" provide advanced practitioner care, and that only "doctors" need be consulted in discussion of that care. This is the case even in areas in which APRNs in fact play a critical role, such as primary care, obstetric care, and public health.

A striking example of the absent APRN is Deirdre Kennedy's April 2008 National Public Radio report about the expanding use of online "doctor-patient" communication. As is typical, the five-minute piece referred relentlessly to "doctors," as if the quarter of a million U.S. APRNs did not exist. But nursing did get one disdainful mention: At one point, Kennedy noted that some "doctors" were using a physician-designed Web portal that asked patients preliminary questions about their conditions, using "branching logic." Kennedy referred to this computer system as an "electronic advice nurse."

When news items do discuss APRN care, they may indicate that APRNs are poor substitutes for physicians. Many pieces rely for expert comment solely on physicians, who often present their assumptions that APRNs can't handle serious conditions because they have not been educated as physicians. Many such reports do not even give APRNs the chance to respond to uninformed attacks on the care they give. Here again, it must be enough to just "ask your doctor"!

Sometimes physicians themselves create such media. An August 2008 *Washington Post* piece by physician Benjamin Natelson bemoaned the decline in physicians' ability and willingness to make difficult diagnoses, which the author attributes mainly to modern health care economics. Natelson writes that a "partial solution to the growing gap in primary care providers" is "physician extenders," who are "trained to deal with commonly occurring, easy-to-diagnose problems: a flu, hay fever, a splinter, even severe chest pain." However, he claims, these "extenders" usually have not "had enough training to give them the know-how to sort through a complex medical history to arrive at a diagnosis that isn't immediately evident. When they're stuck, they have to call the physician, and by then, the 30-minute visit is very often over." Natelson wrongly conflates years of formal education with the ability to diagnose, and diagnosis with all of health care, as in *House.* In fact, NPs have used their advanced listening skills to diagnose many life-threatening conditions that physicians did not. But more generally, NPs achieve good patient outcomes because they are adept at the full range of what practitioners should do, including preventative health and patient education. Ironically, another NP asset is just what Natelson disdains: NPs' willingness to consult with others when they do not know. Plus, with those graduate science degrees, NPs are super at splinters!

Sometimes reporters rely on physicians in conveying baseless disrespect for APRNs, often providing no opportunity for APRNs to respond. A November 2002 *Redbook* article entitled "Advice Docs Give Their Own Families" included a physician warning: "Don't let yourself be brushed off onto a Nurse Practitioner."

Nurse anesthetists have received special attention from high-end plastic surgeons in the media. Some surgeons advise patients that CRNAs are unsafe, though a great deal of research shows the opposite to be true. In June 2004 *Vogue* ran a piece by Ariel Levy about cosmetic surgery that quoted Santa Monica surgeon R. Patrick Abergel, whose patients include Hollywood stars, as follows: "It's not illegal for surgeons to administer anesthesia themselves, and a lot do — or they work with nurse anesthetists. Both are unsafe." We can't help but wonder if elite plastic surgeons who denigrate CRNAs tend to justify their high fees in part through their own association with anesthesiologists, essentially a type of medical upselling.

Coverage of the growth in the number of clinics based in U.S. supermarkets and drugstores rarely conveys much respect for NPs. A July 2006 *Houston Chronicle* report, Brett Brune's "In-store Clinics Not a Cure-all, Doctors Warn," describes the American Medical Association's efforts to limit the rapid expansion of retail clinics. Physician Michael Speer of the Texas Medical Association allows that the idea of the clinics has "some degree of merit" for things like flu shots, simple abrasions, colds, and other "minor illnesses." But he suggests that (in the reporter's words) "if stitches are needed or a cough gets deeper, it's time to go to a doctor." The *Chronicle*'s main source on NP skill is AMA board member Dr. Rebecca Patchin, who at the time was using her status as a "former nurse" to bolster misleading press attacks on NPs in retail clinics. In the *Chronicle*, Patchin says the AMA wants

> to make sure the public understands when it's appropriate to use a store-based clinic and when they should utilize an emergency room or a doctor's office.... When I was a nurse, I didn't know as much as I know now.... The extra years of training as a physician provide added experience, exposure and depth of knowledge regarding patients, illness, disease process and treatment.

But this is not a fair comparison of NPs and MDs because Patchin was never an NP. Patchin also asserts that physicians (in Brune's words) "have at least five more years of education than nurse practitioners." This formulation wrongly equates NPs' undergraduate education, which includes two years of health care training, with physicians' undergraduate education, which does not. It also wrongly counts physician residencies as education but not the early years of NP practice, or the many years of RN practice that most NPs have. And like all who claim that NPs are unsafe, Patchin ignores the research showing the contrary.

In an apparent stab at balance, the *Chronicle* piece includes reaction from a retail clinic company CEO. He says that most customers have no primary care provider but that they are discouraged from making the clinics their "medical home" for anything other than "routine episodic care." Of course quick clinics should be clear about their scope of care. But like most comments by retail clinic executives in similar articles, this one does not convey that NPs are skilled professionals who can themselves provide comprehensive primary care in a setting that allows for it. There is no recognition that the type of vaccinations and basic screenings the retail clinics provide have saved millions of lives around the world. No NP is consulted for the piece, suggesting that physicians are the only health experts with anything useful to say about NP care. And there is no hint that the rise of retail-based clinics can be viewed not just as a clever business initiative, but as a promising new basic care model.

Similarly, in November 2005 NBC's popular *Today* show included a short, troubling segment about the retail clinics by reporter Janice Lieberman. While stressing that the clinics offer convenience and affordability for basic care, the report also degraded the NP care available "on the cheap" at what it called "quickie" clinics. It ignored

NPs' vital role in more comprehensive primary care, and suggested that autonomous NP care presents safety risks, relying on a quote about the supposed need for "supervision" of the "non-physician providers" from AMA president Edward Hill. The only audible NP response the NBC News product offered its audience consisted of an NP, identified as "Kathy," saying "ready" to indicate that she was set to give Lieberman a flu shot.

Some news items praise APRNs in a way that denigrates non-APRN RNs, at times based on comment from APRNs themselves. The April 2008 *Wall Street Journal* piece about the development of the DNP degree included a chart comparing the education and practice of DNPs, master's-prepared APRNs, and RNs. Under the heading of "Professional Authority," the chart listed the APRNs' prescription authority; for the RNs, it stated "None." Nonsense. RNs cannot prescribe drugs, but that does not mean they have no authority, as the nurse practice acts discussed in chapter 4 make clear.

In February 2005 the *Australian* ran a good piece by Adam Cresswell about the growing role of Australian NPs in managing chronic heart failure. "The rise of the super nurse" emphasizes the positive effect of the holistic nursing model on patient outcomes. But the term "super nurse," even more than "advanced practice nurse," may suggest that RNs are nothing special.

Similarly, a January–February 2005 issue of *U.S. News & World Report* featured a massive special health report, consisting of many smaller pieces, entitled "Who Needs Doctors?" Describing how other professionals are increasingly providing care that used to be the exclusive province of physicians, the report takes an unusually positive look at the work of APRNs. Some parts of the report suggest, however, that APRNs are worthy of attention because they're doing things physicians do, whereas other nurses remain engaged in their subservient, limited traditional work. One NP is quoted as saying that when she started out (in about 1980) "nurses were not told we could think for ourselves" and "just did what a doctor planned out for us," which is incorrect. Some nurses may have (wrongly) internalized the idea that they have not been thinking for themselves, but autonomous thinking has been a critical part of nursing practice since at least Nightingale's time, as we discuss in chapter 4. The feature states that "through the 1980's, the idea of nurses doing more than just assisting doctors gained acceptance" as patients began seeking out nurses as their primary care providers. The statement obviously implies that RNs simply assist physicians, which we know is false. For centuries, nursing has been an autonomous science profession with its own distinct sphere of practice, even though it has had less power than medicine.

Thus, even in many APRN pieces, a troubling theme remains: Now that APRNs can do work that physicians have been doing, who needs RNs?

# PART 3

# Seeking Better Understanding of Nursing — and Better Health Care

CHAPTER 10

# How We Can All Improve Understanding of Nursing

O NE AFTERNOON WE DROVE in the drizzling rain along the winding Rock Creek Parkway in Washington, DC. Suddenly we saw a commotion ahead. A car had just slid off the road and flipped upside down. A small crowd had gathered, but paramedics had not yet arrived. We stopped, and Sandy got out to help, having practiced emergency nursing at major trauma centers for many years.

Sandy approached the overturned car. The driver was suspended upside down by her seat belt. She was conscious but understandably anxious. A group of about ten people, mostly men, was frantically trying to figure out how to remove the driver from her car. Sandy spoke loudly: "I'm a nurse. Do you need help?" The crowd ignored Sandy and continued preparing to move the woman. If the woman had had a serious neck injury, moving her without immobilization precautions could have caused paralysis or even death, so Sandy said loudly, "Is anyone else here a health professional?" Again no one replied. So Sandy said, "OK then, I'm an ER nurse, I'm in charge here."

Very reluctantly, the crowd gave Sandy enough room — barely — to push through to examine the upside-down patient. A few men in the crowd demanded that Sandy let them get the woman out. Sandy assessed the woman's neck and general condition. She had no apparent serious injury, so Sandy let the crowd take her down.

Every day, people in situations like this depend on nurses to advocate for them. But in this case, as in many others, the nurse was barely able to protect the patient. It's hard to escape the conclusion that this danger arises from the public's misunderstanding of nursing. The crowd at Rock Creek conveyed confusion, even anger, that a nurse would purport to direct them on a life-threatening health condition, even though no one else present had health expertise. Perhaps the crowd, like surgeon character Cristina Yang on *Grey's Anatomy*, would have been happy to let Sandy know if a bedpan needed emptying! But if Sandy had announced that she was a physician, it is hard to imagine the same reaction.

We have shown how the media reinforces the undervaluation of nursing. In 2006 a Brazilian nursing professor wrote us to say that she shared our concerns about the popular show *House*, which airs in Brazil and around the world. The professor said nursing was very different in Brazil, because "we don't have to report to doctors; I report to the manager nurse." Of course, U.S. nurses also report to senior nurses, not to physicians. But *House* and other Hollywood shows offer a persuasive enough vision of U.S. health roles that even the nursing professor believed the inaccuracy.

We have also seen that public disrespect for nursing has grave consequences for nurses and patients. Disrespect underlies many of the more immediate causes of the deadly nursing shortage. It leads governments and foundations to allot meager funding for nursing education and research. That in turn undermines the nursing profession, leaving too few qualified nurses and nursing educators, and people die. We rightly spend billions on alleviating deadly diseases, but we spend relatively little on the poor nursing infrastructure that allows the diseases to spread in the first place. Disrespect leads hospital administrators to replace RNs with technicians, who can't tell when a patient is deteriorating, so patients die. Disrespect leads patients to ignore nurses' health teaching, and the patients may die. Disrespect undermines nurses' sense of their own worth, deterring them from advocating for themselves and their patients.

We can change this situation. Poor public understanding of nursing, and the resulting harm to public health, is not inevitable. Of course changing the way the world thinks is a challenge, but even the most ingrained social biases can change over time. And nurses have already managed to improve understanding, in ways large and small. Nurses have persuaded or helped some media creators to produce more accurate news articles and even entertainment media. Nurses have convinced advertisers to reconsider degrading naughty nurse depictions. We've seen how in 2005 nurses persuaded the U.S. government to change the name of the Take a Loved One to the Doctor Day campaign to Take a Loved One for a Checkup Day, a name that does not exclude the APRNs who provide primary care to the minority populations the campaign targets.

But understanding does not improve only through media products that reach millions. All of us can have a powerful effect simply by the way we think and act every day. Sandy was raised in a family with a strong focus on mechanical and computer science, but she considered nursing to be undesirable handmaiden work until, as a teenager, she worked at a nursing home. She was awed by the skill and autonomy she saw in the nurses there. She began nursing school. Not all nurses would have inspired that choice. That these nurses did is a testament to their professional strength and vision.

*Everyone* should play a role in increasing understanding of nursing. Of course nurses must take the lead, as we'll discuss in detail in chapter 11. Nurses should learn that what the media says and the public thinks about their profession matters. Nurses' poor working conditions and lack of resources are a direct result of what powerful decision makers really think of them. Nurses have a duty to advocate for patients, and that requires more respect than nursing now has. Nurses must believe in themselves and project that belief to others. Nurses should persuade the media to provide a more accurate picture of the profession, and they should consider creating new media themselves.

But nurses cannot improve understanding by themselves, because they are underpowered, even in their own spheres of expertise. Few nurses serve as hospital CEOs or as directors on hospital boards, even though hospitals exist mainly to provide nursing care. Few nurses hold powerful positions in government or the private sector. Few nurses have significant input on influential media.

Many other segments of society can help nurses by influencing both media portrayals of nursing and people's understanding of nursing generally. We can all listen to nurses and watch what actually happens when we interact with the health care system: What are the nurses doing? Does the media we see reflect that? Tell a friend! What are our assumptions and actions when it comes to nursing, including our language; do we credit physicians for things nurses really do? And how can we apply our new understanding to push for more resources and respect for the skilled nurses almost all of us will one day need?

Some parts of society have special influence. In particular, those who create media should try harder to provide a fair picture of nursing. Creators of news and entertainment media can learn from nurses about what they really do. And nurses make great expert sources, because they are trained to convey their knowledge to lay people. In addition, advertisers should consider the effects of nursing stereotypes and try to find alternative ways to sell their products.

Private sector health executives should ensure that their public speech reflects an understanding of nursing. Hospital managers should promote nursing as they do medicine, and publicize their efforts to strengthen the profession. Insurers and drug companies can advertise without suggesting that health care revolves solely around "doctors."

Government leaders and other health policy makers should also work to communicate an understanding of what nurses really do. They should publicize their efforts to invest in nurses' clinical practice, education, and research, and place qualified nurses in visible positions of authority. Foundations should consider creating prizes and museums to build public appreciation for nursing.

Nurses' health care colleagues can also play a key role. Physicians must learn about what nurses really do for patients, and they should work to stop the crediting of physicians for nurses' work, from Hollywood to your bedside. Other health workers should ensure that they are not mistaken for nurses.

What will the future look like when the global public truly values the nursing profession? *Understanding that nurses save lives will itself save lives* — by providing the resources and respect nurses need to do their work. Adequate resources for clinical settings are only the beginning. Through their holistic, preventative focus, nurses can intervene before conditions become severe, so that patients don't end up dead or in expensive hospitals. Teams consisting of community health nurses and advanced practice nurses, working in local settings, can prevent or manage a great deal of the illness the world now suffers. With such programs, malaria might kill millions fewer children, because the nurse teams could work to eliminate standing pools of water and increase use of mosquito nets. Obesity-related problems like heart disease and diabetes might no longer cripple health systems if nurses were educating and advocating in the community for better diet and exercise. Millions of critically ill infants might be home with their families because nurses would have the resources to teach mothers how and why to breastfeed. Emergency departments might no longer burst with patients waiting twenty hours for care, because nurses would be keeping many patients out of the hospital system.

Here is a prospectus for a global investment in nursing:

Value of nurses saving thousands of additional lives every day:
Trillions of dollars.

Value of nurses teaching millions more people how to live healthier lives:
Trillions of dollars.

Value of nurses keeping families, workplaces, communities, and nations strong:
Priceless.

Everyone can do *something* to increase knowledge of what nurses really do and thereby improve health. Below are some ideas, conveniently organized for specific categories of people. Clip 'n' save!

# I'M A CITIZEN OF THE WORLD. WHAT CAN I DO?

We can all learn more about nursing — what it is and is not. When you are in the health care system, or meet a nurse, try to learn what nurses really do. We can all look critically at what the media tells us about nursing. Does that news story or show treat nursing fairly? If not, is that acceptable in the midst of a nursing crisis? We can all consider the messages that we ourselves send, through things as basic as our clothes and our language. What each of us does matters particularly now, because with the Internet, virtually anyone can create media accessible to the rest of the world, all day, every day.

## "What do you do all day, anyway?"

When you meet a nurse, try asking what was exciting or worthwhile about the care he or she provided to patients in recent days. Try to focus on what the nurse actually did for the patient: How did he improve the patient's outcome? Did she save (or lose) a life? The nurse will get a chance to practice explaining what nursing involves and perhaps gain reassurance that it matters. And you'll probably learn something new about nursing.

## "You could be a doctor!"

Let's say a nurse tells you a fascinating story and you are floored by his skilled, autonomous interventions. (Stay with us, this often happens when people really listen.) Try to resist the urge to tell him, "You could be a doctor!" We know that people mean this as a compliment, but it suggests that any health care worker who displays knowledge or skill must be destined to be a physician, since nurses do not have or need such qualities. When a specific nurse does, many people understandably conclude that she must be exceptional. In fact, knowledge-able, skilled nurses are not the exception but the rule.

## Don't Believe the Hype

We can all look more critically at what the media presents to us. The next time the news media consults only physicians for a story about something in which nurses are expert, like hospital conditions, consider why nurses were ignored — and what the story is not telling you as a result. Research shows that even the entertainment media affects our thinking, as we explained in chapter 2. So when a hospital drama shows physicians providing all skilled hospital care, ask yourself how likely that is. Would nurses be providing much of that care? Ask media creators why they do not give a fair account of nursing. It's fun!

## Try to Resist That Naughty Nurse's Charms

Naughty nurse pornography, lingerie, and costumes remain popular, though they reinforce a tired, damaging stereotype. Sexual fantasies cannot be simply wished away, but we can consider new ways to think about nurses. And we urge those who profit from naughty nurse products to consider other ways to prosper.

Say you're invited to a Halloween party. You could wear some naughty nurse costume. But the naughty nurse really is a corpse bride, because she scares away the resources nurses need to save lives. So consider telling some other tale from the crypt.

## Name That Provider

Language is powerful. Unfortunately, too many common words and phrases reinforce damaging assumptions and stereotypes about nursing. Many of these usages degrade nurses' professional identity or credit others for their work. Of course, purposely changing language is difficult, but you can start with yourself. You may expand your mind — and improve your health. The table below outlines ten troubling usages and suggests alternatives.

| Common word or phrase | Better words or phrases | Why consider the change? |
|---|---|---|
| angel | nurse | When we refer to nurses as "angels," we imply that they are unskilled spiritual beings who don't need good salaries, rest, or resources. "Angels" can take care of ten patients on their mandatory sixteen-hour shifts and never make a serious mistake. Humans can't. |
| baby nurse | newborn nanny or caregiver | Many people refer to infant caregivers as "baby nurses," but these workers do not have a nursing education, and most have little or no health education. |
| doctor | physician | Using "doctor" to describe only physicians elevates them above other health workers and gives the false impression that physicians are the only health workers who earn doctoral degrees. |
| medical center | hospital | Many vital health professionals besides physicians work in hospitals. Yet because only physicians practice "medicine," the term "medical center" suggests hospitals are all about physicians. |

| Common word or phrase | Better words or phrases | Why consider the change? |
|---|---|---|
| medicine (to mean all health care) | health care | Medicine, which physicians practice, is one type of health care, but many others are also important. Health fields like nursing are not subsets of medicine but distinct, autonomous fields. |
| nurse (to mean anyone who provides any care) | nursing assistant, medical technician, or whatever they really are | Only nurses should be called "nurse." When non-nurses are called "nurse," people interacting with them may reasonably conclude that nurses know far less about health care than they really do. Many family members admirably provide care for their loved ones, but this does not make them "nurses." |
| nursing or wet nursing (to mean breastfeeding) | breastfeeding | Using "nursing" or "wet nursing" to mean breastfeeding subtly suggests that nursing is something we can do without health training, and of course that only women can be nurses, which is not the case. |
| order | prescription or care plan | Nurses don't take "orders" from physicians. If nurses do not agree with a physician plan, they are legally and ethically obligated to work for a better plan. |
| she (to refer to a nurse of indefinite gender) | he, or he or she | Some nurses prefer female pronouns, because most nurses are women, and women predominate in few professions. But one way to undermine the prevailing social bias that nurses are all female is to use "he" when discussing nurses of indefinite gender. |

| Common word or phrase | Better words or phrases | Why consider the change? |
|---|---|---|
| "work as a nurse" | "practice nursing" | Nurses are professionals who "practice" nursing, just as physicians practice medicine. Nurses do not stop being nurses when they go home for the day or when they stop providing direct care at the bedside. |

# I'M A MEMBER OF THE MEDIA. WHAT CAN I DO?

As the global population ages, it becomes even more interested in health. If you create media about health care, we urge you to learn all you can about what nurses really do. Whether you work for a newspaper, a website, an ad agency, or Hollywood, please listen to nurses when they point out inaccuracies and distortions. The input will improve your work.

## Report on the Nurse at the Bedside

The bedside nurse saves lives and sees it all, and some reports have given readers a sense of that. But the news media has barely skimmed the surface. Nurses save lives in countless ways, managing high-tech interventions, catching subtle but deadly errors, and spearheading public health programs. And don't forget nursing errors: the media generally assumes that only physician errors matter, but in fact nurses affect patient outcomes just as much, and so their care deserves the same scrutiny. Nurses spend far more time with patients than anyone else, and they see people at their best and their worst. Nursing is vital and exciting. News consumers would be interested in what nurses do and what they know, if only the consumers heard more about it. Be receptive to what nurses tell you, and ask them questions. Too many reporters and editors rely on inaccurate assumptions about nursing, or on physicians, who, sadly, often don't know much about nursing either. Physicians dominate media like the *New York Times* and CNN, creating many stories themselves. But when nurses are given the chance — as in oncology nurse Theresa Brown's powerful September 2008 "Cases" piece in the *Times* — they too can create compelling and informative pieces.

## Discover 2.7 Million Women in Science

There are scientific breakthroughs all the time — and they're published in peer-reviewed nursing journals like the *American Journal of Nursing*. The news media's audience would be interested in many of these, such as the studies about how hospital conditions affect patients, the latest advances in pain control, and innovative health initiatives addressing problems like HIV and diabetes. Nursing should be presented as the cutting-edge health science it is. The media sometimes runs stories about women in science, but these reports typically overlook the 2.7 million female RNs in the United States, including the 350,000 with master's and doctoral degrees. In fact, nurses have long done fascinating, groundbreaking work. The work of nursing pioneers like nurse midwife Mary Breckinridge and public health nurse Lillian Wald remains influential even today. Informing your audience about these nursing pioneers may pique interest in the profession's current leaders.

## Consider Nurses as Expert Sources in All Health Stories

Nurses make great media health experts. They combine advanced health knowledge with the ability to communicate important health ideas to lay people, as part of their focus on patient education.

Unfortunately, nurse experts often struggle to be heard. Some news outlets consult nurses when the topic is some aspect of nursing, such as the nursing shortage. But nurses rarely appear as experts when the topic is health in general. Virtually no hospitals have public relations officials devoted to promoting their nurses in the media, as almost all do for physicians. But Georgia Peirce of Massachusetts General Hospital is one such publicist. When reporters call Peirce looking for an expert, she often suggests a stellar nurse who has expertise in the area of interest. Nevertheless, the reporters usually insist on a physician. When the media doesn't see nurses as experts, and so does not present them that way, the public shares that view. The public does not understand why nursing requires many resources, and it takes nurses' health advice less seriously, in clinical settings and otherwise. The public also comes to see health through a physician-centered lens, as something that involves the diagnosis and treatment of illness. If the media used nurses as expert sources, the public might develop a stronger sense of health as attaining and maintaining wellness. Consulting nurse experts would create richer media, help reshape debates on health, and offer new ideas to repair the broken health care system.

The few media programs that do routinely use nurse experts show how effective the practice can be. One that may use nurse experts more than any other is *HealthStyles*, the weekly radio show on New York's WBAI, hosted by nurses Diana Mason, editor-in-chief of the *American Journal of Nursing*, and Barbara Glickstein. On this show, nurse experts discuss health topics we don't often hear elsewhere, such as the movement in care of the dying from a "do not resuscitate" focus toward plans to "allow a natural death." Nurse Pat Carroll appears on Connecticut television stations to explain health issues. Nurses Barbara Dehn and Nancy Reame appear on iVillage to discuss maternal-child issues.

## Make Clear That Nurse Experts Are Nurses

When nurse experts do appear in media items, their status as nurses is often hidden. When the media identifies an expert as "Dr. Pugh" most people assume the expert is a physician. And even when a nurse expert's PhD is noted, few will realize he or she is a nurse unless the piece says so. The media should identify experts as nurses so that the profession receives credit for the knowledge they provide. Indeed, it is more important for the RN to appear than the "Dr." or the PhD.

## Create TV Shows about Nurses

Though real nursing is dramatic and exciting, few television shows feature nurses as main characters. Instead, they present nurses as peripheral to serious care and focus almost solely on physician characters — who are shown spending much of their time doing what nurses do in real life. There have been some recent exceptions. As we noted in chapter 2, in early 2009 Showtime is scheduled to introduce a half-hour dark comedy about a New York emergency nurse tentatively titled *Nurse Jackie*. And in fall 2008 the travel agency Access Nurses syndicated some of its Web-based *NurseTV* reality programming, which briefly examines real nurses at work and elsewhere, in minor television markets and stations throughout the United States. However, the rarity and limited scope of these exceptions proves the rule.

## But Aren't Hollywood's Current Nurse Advisers Enough?

Nurses do advise many Hollywood shows, like *Grey's Anatomy*, but their main role seems to be teaching the actors playing physicians how to behave credibly on set. Obviously, "nursing advice" that has no evident impact on how the show actually depicts nursing does not help the profession. As with the news media, physicians dominate in providing the advice that drives the story lines. Only meaningful advice on scripts by nurses who understand nursing's media issues can help, and producers must be more open to it.

In chapter 2 we described how a nurse who is an international expert in her specialty recently got a phone call from producers of a popular TV hospital show. After she gave the producers the information they wanted, she tried to educate them about why they should include more nursing in their show. This was a great effort, but not surprisingly this one interaction wasn't enough to change the show. In fact, although the producers were stunned to learn that our friend is a nurse — an expert and a nurse! — they still told her that they and their audience were interested only in physicians.

## But How Can I Sell Things Without Using Nursing Stereotypes?

With imagination, you can advertise your product without resorting to tired and demeaning stereotypes. It's true that the naughty nurse has been an advertising mainstay, and other ads have presented nurses as handmaidens or relatively unskilled. But that need not be so. If advertisers wonder if they are using nursing imagery in a responsible way, they should consult with those familiar with nursing's image issues. Contact us at info@nursingadvocacy.org. We'll help you at no charge! Or take the campaign in a different direction. Advertising professionals can be very creative.

Advertisers do not wish to alienate consumers, and some advertisers have been commendably flexible when nurses bring issues to their attention. Some companies, like Skechers, have curtailed ads that relied so heavily on nursing stereotypes that they could not be salvaged. Others, including Wal-Mart and CVS, have modified ads to eliminate nursing stereotypes, with no apparent loss of effectiveness. For example, in 2007 Heineken brand Dos Equis launched an amusing set of beer ads in a mock-serious tribute to a character presented as "the most interesting man in the world." The ads showed him bench-pressing two chairs in which sat attractive, giggly women in short white dresses with nurses' caps. In response to our concerns, Heineken digitally altered the women's clothing to eliminate the nursing identifiers. We encourage other advertisers to show similar flexibility and imagination.

## "I Wouldn't Stereotype Nurses — My Mom's a Nurse!"

Please don't be one of those media creators who claim that they could not possibly create media that harms nursing because they're related to nurses or just really love nurses. Just as it makes no difference that a nurse was involved in creating a television show if that show harms nursing, it makes no difference that a media creator is close to nurses if his show, ad, or other product stereotypes them. For instance, even though *House* regularly degrades nursing, a show representative once suggested that the show can't harm nursing, in part, because the mother of creator David Shore is a nurse, and she just loves the show! And we have heard from other media creators that their shows couldn't harm nursing because close relatives of the show creators are nurses (as with Dr. Phil) or the creators previously expressed appreciation for nurses (as with David Letterman). But there's no reason to think the *effects* of these shows change because of the relatives or intentions of the creators. We urge media creators to consider whether the images they *actually present* conform with their positive sentiments about nursing.

# I'M A PRIVATE SECTOR HEALTH CARE EXECUTIVE. WHAT CAN I DO?

If you are an executive at a hospital or other organization that provides health care (like the Red Cross or Doctors Without Borders), or at a health insurance company or pharmaceutical company, there is much you can do to help nurses improve understanding of their profession. Whether you realize it or not, you play a key role in shaping how the media treats nursing and how the public sees it.

## Hospitals and Health Facilities Should Promote Nursing

Hospital executives can and should promote nursing to the media and through many other avenues, inside and outside the hospital. Because your facility's nursing is just as important to patient outcomes as its medicine is, nursing deserves the same attention.

Promote nursing within hospital walls, to physicians, to patients, and to the nurses themselves: some may need reminding of their own importance! Tell physicians what their nurse colleagues actually do. Give patients information about what the nurses do and why, the qualifications of your nurses, and the hospital's efforts to strengthen nursing. Help your nurses tell everyone who they are. In today's clinical settings, many different staff wear similar uniforms, and in some cases this trend has obscured efforts to replace nurses with cheaper unlicensed personnel. Instead, facilities should encourage nurses to wear distinctive uniforms and use other identifiers, like RN patches. That way, nurses receive the credit and blame they deserve, and understanding of their true role in heath care grows.

### INVEST IN PUBLIC RELATIONS FOR NURSING

Every hospital should have a public relations professional to promote the facility's nurses, their stories, research, and community activities, and to direct media inquiries to nurses when their expertise is called for. Yet we know of only two hospitals that have a PR officer who works solely on promoting the nursing profession.

Georgia Peirce is the PR person for nursing at Massachusetts General Hospital (MGH). She is not a nurse, but she persuaded the *Boston Globe* to follow nurses in the hospital and to create one of the best newspaper accounts of nursing practice that we have seen in the last decade. The result was the excellent four-part October 2005 series about MGH ICU nurses, especially a formidable veteran who was training a new nurse, as described in chapters 3 and 4. Reporter Scott Allen and photographer Michele McDonald followed the nurses intermittently for nine months. Their series, which remains available online, educates society about the vital, skilled, and difficult work that nurses do.

To make the *Globe* series happen, Peirce spent time picking the right medium and the right writer. She geared her pitch around a high-autonomy area for nursing, the ICU. She focused on nurses in a mentor/apprentice role, so that it would be easier for the reporter to learn what was going on inside their heads. That might otherwise have been difficult, because nurses are still socialized to defer and mask their skills. It took Peirce three weeks to overcome the *Globe*'s skepticism, but after she persuaded the reporter to come observe, he found plenty of interest and he agreed to pursue the story.

## Publicize Efforts to Improve Nurses' Working Conditions

If you're an executive at a health care institution during today's nursing crisis, you probably want to improve the morale of your nursing staff and reduce turnover. The best way to do that is to strengthen nursing. Reversing the denursification of health care can save hospitals money and save patients' lives. But if you publicize what you're doing — as many hospitals have publicized their Magnet status — through advertising and other media, you can also improve understanding of nursing. You will not only present your institution in a positive light but also explain nursing to society and encourage others to take similar steps. Specific ideas to consider include

- increasing RN-to-patient ratios, eliminating the use of "techs" for nursing tasks;

- helping nurses improve their education levels, including through tuition reimbursement, and providing rigorous continuing education and professional development programs;

- empowering nurses by including them in authoritative positions and roles, including on your governing board, ethics committees, morbidity and mortality conferences, patient-family meetings, and nurse-driven daily rounds;

- creating multi-year nursing residencies;

- providing nurses with far more support staff, including aides and clerks;

- ensuring that each unit has 24/7 coverage by clinical nurse specialists; and

- instituting zero tolerance for abuse policies.

There are many more suggestions on the Center's website at nursingadvocacy.org/faq/magnet.html. If you implement changes like these, tell the world: you're helping to resolve the nursing crisis.

## Public Health Organizations Can Help Promote Nursing

Nurses play central roles in some of the most respected and well-known non-governmental health institutions, and it is vital that these institutions convey respect for nursing as well. Some could do far more. For instance, in mid-2008 the American Red Cross announced to the public — 127 years after nurse Clara Barton founded the organization — that it was eliminating its chief nursing officer position as part of budget cutbacks. Or consider the Nobel Prize–winning Médecins Sans Frontières (MSF) or Doctors Without Borders. This international aid group was founded by a small group of physicians and journalists, but today more nurses than physicians work for MSF, and nurses have played leadership roles in the group. Yet its name sends the public the message that the physicians provide most or all of its health care. That message is especially influential because the group receives tremendous media attention for its work on disasters worldwide. Nursing advocates have asked MSF to consider a more inclusive name, such as Soins Sans Frontières (Health Care Without Borders). So far, MSF has refused.

## Health Insurers

Health insurance companies and the health institutions they reimburse should keep the nursing out of the mashed potatoes. Nursing care should be billed and reimbursed as a professional service, just like the work of physicians and others. Currently, skilled nursing care does not appear on U.S. hospital bills as a distinct item but is instead included in "room and board" charges. When nursing is lumped in with the bedsheets and hospital food, people are encouraged to see nurses as interchangeable widgets, not professionals. Early nurses provided the full range of care that patients needed, including physical therapy, occupational therapy, speech-language therapy, and social work. Over time these fields became separate professions, most of which now bill independently for their work. Nursing is no less skilled. Allowing nurses to bill separately would open up a dialogue that would force decision makers, the media, and the public to learn about and articulate the nature of nursing work.

## Drug Companies Should Ask Their Nurses

As we all know, advertising for medications and other health care products typically advises consumers to "ask your doctor" whether the product is right for them. This phrase obviously assumes that only physicians have expertise in such products and prescription authority, but neither of those ideas is correct. Nurses, especially advanced practice nurses, are the primary care providers for millions of health consumers, and these tremendously influential ad campaigns should recognize that. In 2008 the American Academy of Nurse Practitioners began a campaign to persuade pharmaceutical companies to change the language in their commercials to "ask your provider."

As health products makers, drug companies also have a special responsibility to advertise in a way that recognizes the contributions of the nurses who actually administer most of their products in hospital settings. In 2006 a Bristol Myers–Squibb television commercial featured Sharon Blynn reciting a poem on fighting cancer that included the line "Doctors who tell jokes in the chemo room are beautiful." However, virtually all chemo room work is done by nurses. And though Johnson & Johnson deserves credit for putting tens of millions of dollars into its campaign to help resolve the nursing shortage, as we have explained in previous chapters, it should also work to reduce its heavy reliance on damaging angel and handmaiden imagery. Like hospitals, influential drug companies can enhance their own images by promoting nursing, but in doing so they should learn and communicate that nurses are highly skilled professionals who save lives and improve patient outcomes.

# I'M A GOVERNMENT OR HEALTH POLICY MAKER. WHAT CAN I DO?

We urge government and health policy makers to learn the value of nursing and convey their knowledge wherever they can. They should publicize the urgency of the nursing shortage and their efforts to address it, which will tell the public that nursing has value. And major foundations should consider funding various initiatives to improve understanding of nursing, including prizes, museums, and popular media programming.

## Governments Should Communicate the Value of Nursing

The government has great power to direct the flow of information to the media and the public. Government leaders should use that power to convey the true nature and importance of nursing. They should appoint qualified nurses to visible positions of authority, as President Bill Clinton did in choosing nurse Kristine Gebbie as the first "AIDS czar" in 1993. Public health campaigns are also useful in getting the word out.

One notable recent idea is nurse Teri Mills's proposal to establish an Office of the National Nurse within the U.S. Public Health Service. The main purposes of the National Nurse would be to promote public health through media-driven preventative health education and the deployment of community health nurses, and to highlight for the public the key role that nurses play and the threat posed by the nursing shortage. This initiative has been introduced in Congress, and it would appear to offer a promising way to increase public understanding of the profession.

## Governments Should Publicize Efforts to Address the Shortage

Government and other health policy leaders at all levels should communicate their efforts to support nursing and address the nursing shortage. That would not only attract support for the initiatives of these leaders but also highlight the importance of nursing and inspire the private sector to follow suit. Specific improvements that public sector health leaders should consider include

- investing far more in nursing education, clinical practice, and research, since nursing currently gets only a tiny fraction of the government resources that medicine does;
- passing minimum nurse staffing legislation to address the denursification of clinical settings, as well as to limit mandatory overtime and provide whistle-blower protection;
- vastly increasing funding for community health nursing projects such as school nurses and nurse-family partnerships, which would enhance health and educate the public about nursing; and
- making it a major public priority to resolve the nursing shortage, including the formation of working groups and policy discussion at the highest levels.

Leaders should regularly address these issues in their interactions with the media.

## Foundations and Other Health Policy Makers Should Honor Nursing

Major foundations should consider bold initiatives that could radically change the way the media and the public sees nursing. In a 2006

*Baltimore Sun* op-ed, Sandy and Kristine Gebbie argued that nurses deserve a Nobel Prize or comparable annual award. We noted that nursing leaders have long been at the forefront of health research and clinical practice, reinventing health systems, pioneering new therapies, and improving community health, from AIDS treatment to neonatal care. The Nobel Prize in Nursing would shine a light on the profession's achievements and help show how important it is that nursing get the resources it needs to overcome the global shortage.

Foundations should also consider creating an International Museum of Modern Nursing to educate the public about nursing. We envision an interactive science museum that would show that nursing is an exciting profession whose members use the latest technologies to help people regain and maintain health, and that nurse scholars work on the cutting edge of health research. Visitors would be invited to put themselves in the place of nurses on the front lines, in settings ranging from the extreme high-tech of teaching hospital ICUs to humanitarian relief projects around the world.

Foundations should also consider funding television shows and educational materials about nursing, including documentaries and scripted dramas. We envision realistic, engaging depictions of nurses at work, to show nursing as a skilled field in which men and women save lives. Foundations might also consider creating videos to educate the media, physicians, career seekers, and students about nursing.

Foundations and health policy makers should include nurses in advisory groups. In 2007 Google created a Health Advisory Council[1] with twenty-five members, and though many were physicians, not a single one appeared to be a nurse. The powerful media company refused requests to place nurses on the panel. Health initiatives like this cannot succeed without the input of nurses. And of course, including nurses in such high-profile positions would tell the public that nurses are health experts whose work has value.

## I'M A HEALTH WORKER BUT NOT A NURSE. WHAT CAN I DO?

Nurses' health care colleagues, particularly physicians, can help nurses improve public understanding.

### Physicians

Physicians wield unmatched authority over how the media presents health care and how the public sees it. Unfortunately, much of the worst media about nurses, such as Hollywood dramas, is created in collaboration with physicians. Physicians write for and advise television shows, and they consult on many media programs and news articles. It's no shock that these media generally show little interest in nursing, but the collaborating physicians often cause or allow the media to give physicians credit for the work that nurses really do, and to present nurses as low-skilled physician subordinates.

We need physicians to try to understand nursing better. It appears that few physicians learn much about what nurses really do. With only common social and professional stereotypes to go on, many physicians wrongly assume they are "in charge" of nurses and nursing care. One promising way to improve physicians' understanding is through shadowing programs and other structured interactions during their training. Dartmouth's medical school and hospital have a joint program in which medical students shadow nurses for six lengthy sessions. The students ask nurses questions and meet later to discuss what they have learned. As Ellen Ceppetelli, the nursing co-director of the program, said, "You cannot collaborate with people unless you see them as competent."[2]

## Medical Technicians and Nursing Assistants

Some health care personnel who are not nurses allow patients to call them nurses, and some even call themselves nurses. The result is that nurses lose control of their image. Only those whose title includes "nurse" should call themselves nurses.

## Receptionists and Appointment Clerks

Personnel who provide support to health professionals play a role in shaping how nurses are perceived. Some ask patients, "Would you like an appointment with Dr. Kumwenda or with Eve, our nurse practitioner?" Please refer to advanced practice nurses with honorifics if you do the same for physicians. In this example, you might call Eve "Dr. Peyton" if she has a doctoral degree, or "Nurse Practitioner Peyton" if she does not.

Using the ideas in this chapter, nurses' colleagues and supporters can help increase understanding of the profession and help nurses get the resources they need to resolve the nursing crisis and meet the health challenges of the twenty-first century.

# CHAPTER 11

# How Nurses Can Improve
# Their Own Image

IN ORDER FOR UNDERSTANDING of nursing to improve, nurses and nursing students must exert more influence on their own image. They must educate society and the media about what nurses really do and why it matters, so that the profession can attract the resources and respect it needs to resolve the nursing crisis. No one else can do this — nurses are the key.

The first hurdle in this advocacy is self-image. Some nurses will need to focus first on believing in their own profession, and in their power to effect meaningful change for it. Then nurses should consider ways they can project a professional image in their everyday interactions, from the way they act to the way they dress. Nurses will then be ready to analyze and change the media. Nurses should learn ways to improve how the media portrays nursing. And nurses should consider how to create their own media, to tell the public directly why nursing deserves respect and support.

There is often more than one way to see a given issue or media product. Naturally, some people disagree with us about certain things. We appreciate hearing their perspective, and sometimes they persuade us to change our minds. But even if you disagree with us on some points, we urge you to join us when you agree. Nurses must find common ground and work together, because it's the only way we'll effect change.

## YOU HAVE THE POWER

After many decades of damaging media and social disrespect, improving nursing's image will not be easy. But it must be done. The first thing is to believe that it *can* be done, and more basically, to believe in nursing. Nurses have the power to change the way society sees their profession.

### Take Credit for Your Life-Saving Work

Nurses must take credit for the value of their work. We're not saying nurses should become braggarts, but too many nurses don't even seem to respect their own profession. It appears that some nurses have internalized negative views of themselves and that they may be expressing their frustration at their position in the one acceptable direction: at each other. Many nurses tell reverential stories about their physician colleagues, but not about nurses. Trust us — physicians don't need your help. Nurses save lives every day too. Until it's clear that people understand that, nurses should make sure they do. If you don't want credit for your own work, seek it for your nurse colleagues. To this end, we created a bumper sticker that says "Save Lives. Be a Nurse." It is a recruitment message, but it also tells the public something too few people know. Is it boasting? Whatever. If you send us a stamped envelope, we'll send you a bumper sticker.

## Take Responsibility

The media generally suggests that physicians are responsible for all of health care, including errors. Some articles blame physicians for the errors nurses make. Many nurses seem happy to let this go. But these pieces suggest that nurses are marginal players who report to physicians; they undermine the sense of nursing as an autonomous profession with its own legal and ethical duties. To be seen as true professionals, nurses must accept credit when things go well and responsibility when things do not.

## Take the Lead

Some believe that we can rely on others to fix problems within nursing. Some have actually suggested to us that physicians or their professional groups will lead the way. But the troubling role physicians have played so far in media about nursing suggests that is extremely unlikely. Of course, physicians and others can help nurses improve their image, as discussed in chapter 10, but *nurses* must lead the way.

## Your Voice — Yes, Just Yours — Can Make a Critical Difference

One nurse can change the world. When OR nurse Francine Brock of Placentia, California, visited Las Vegas in 2006, she saw IGT's Nurse Follies slot machine, which features naughty nurse and battle-axe imagery. She wrote to Wynn Las Vegas. The casino quickly began converting its eight to ten Nurse Follies slot machines to another theme, at a cost of $2,000 per machine. Of course, not every change can be made this way. But if you believe in the power of your voice, so might others.

# PROJECTING A PROFESSIONAL IMAGE EVERY DAY

Not to freak you out or anything, but everything you do reflects on the nursing profession. Of course no nurse can be expected to carry that burden 24/7, but we urge you to consider how your everyday actions affect how nurses are viewed.

## Accentuate the Positive: Promoting Nursing in Hard Times

Working conditions for most nurses across the globe are difficult now. But however understaffed and overworked you may be, building up the profession will require nurses to speak highly of it. When talking to non-nurses about nursing, try to show how you've made a positive difference in someone's life through your work. Recall the story in chapter 6 about the Chicago artist who told two nurses that she was sad about the downward trajectory of her daughter's career aspirations, from medicine to nursing, during her childhood. Sandy was one of the nurses. Sandy's nurse friend was speechless. But when there was an opportunity, Sandy said, "You know, there's this perception in society that being a nurse is less valuable than being a physician, but that's actually not true," and she went on to describe some of the things nurses do to help patients live better lives. The artist began to learn about nursing. Increasing understanding of nursing begins with you teaching the person in front of you.

## Introduce Yourself as a Nurse

Many nurses introduce themselves to patients and colleagues as "Jenny," or not at all. This sure is friendly, but sadly, it can also undermine respect for nurses. You don't need to be formal and cold to convey that you are a serious professional. Consider this: "Hi, Ms. Jones. My name is Rich Kimball. I'll be your registered nurse until seven A.M. If you have any problems or questions about your illness or your care, just ask for me, and I will help you, OK?"

## Who Put Cartoon Characters All Over My Uniform?

Nurses should consider whether their uniforms convey that they are professionals. When nurses wore caps, patients could identify them. But caps were annoying and carried deadly infections, so most nurses ditched them in the 1980s. Now many bedside positions are filled by far less educated personnel, and everyone dresses in scrubs. Patients don't know who is who, or who can answer their questions. We love Hello Kitty and SpongeBob Squarepants, but not on nursing uniforms. In 2006 host Matt Lauer of the *Today Show* remarked that nurses "look like they're going on vacation" in their scrubs.[1] Physician Patricia Raymond published a 2004 piece in the *Sacramento Bee* respectfully chastising nurses: "You're the only thing between [your] patients and death, and you're covered in cartoons." Some institutions have gone back to all-white nurse uniforms. While we applaud the effort to reclaim a professional image, white uniforms often evoke the unhelpful angel image discussed in chapter 7. Also, people often use chlorine bleach on whites, which degrades the environment that nurses should protect for their patients. In addition, some men do not favor all-white outfits, and it is vital that nursing not create additional barriers to increasing the number of men in nursing.

Nurses' uniforms should also make clear that nurses are nurses. In 2004 both the *Pittsburgh Post-Gazette* and the *Kansas City Star* ran articles focusing on patients' right to know who is providing their care. To address this problem, we support the RN patch created by J. Morgan Puett and Mark Dion as part of a 2004 exhibit on nursing uniforms at the Fabric Workshop and Museum in Philadelphia. In her personal capacity, Sandy has worked with a uniform maker to create a new line of uniforms to help nurses look more professional. For more information see www.nursingvision.org.[2]

When Texas nurse practitioner Margaret Helminiak accepted a new job, the business manager of the practice offered to buy her scrubs "like we do for the medical assistants." She politely thanked him, but declined: "No, I don't wear scrubs. I didn't go to school for eight years to be mistaken for one of the medical assistants." Helminiak wears a lab coat with "Nurse Practitioner" embroidered on it.

## Nursing Out Loud

Nursing is more about thinking than it is about busy hands. But society doesn't realize it when nurses keep all their thinking to themselves. Because of what Suzanne Gordon has termed the "virtue script," nurses have historically disavowed credit for their work. But to borrow Vice President Dick Cheney's famous remark about conservation, nursing modesty "may be a sign of personal virtue, but it is not a sufficient basis for a sound, comprehensive [public] policy." It will not educate society about nursing. Unlike physicians, nurses cannot count on the assumption that they are *thinking*.

So consider nursing out loud. We don't just mean asserting yourself with colleagues when patient advocacy requires. Patients, families, and colleagues would learn far more about nursing if nurses would describe more of what they are thinking. ("Ms. Keating, when I listen to your lungs, they sound like they are half-filled with fluid. You probably know this is related to your congestive heart failure, but I'm concerned that the fluid is decreasing your oxygen level. Are you having difficulty breathing?") When nurses think out loud, consistent with patient confidentiality and sensitivity, others get a sense of nurses' training and skill. Rhea Sanford, RN, PhD, suggests that if nursing students and new nurses practice out loud, they can "transfer classroom knowledge into quality clinical practice" and assess their own performance, while "providing needed education to their patients."[3]

## Walk the Walk

Nurses live stressful lives, and understandably, some cope in unhealthy ways. Unfortunately, unhealthy behavior may undermine the public's sense of nurses as health professionals. Some nurses have a difficult relationship with food. When nurses become over-weight, patients and the public may doubt their credibility on any health issue, not just nutritional issues. If you need help attaining a healthy weight, consider an easy plan we put together to help you at www.nursingadvocacy.org/action/eating_healthy.html. It is also important to get enough exercise and try to stop smoking. If you exercise, you can teach exercise principles and motivating techniques to your patients. And patients may see nurses who smoke as something other than serious health professionals.

## Act for Change

When nurses are off duty, their actions still say something about nursing. We urge nurses to consider acting as a health resource for their families, friends, and communities. Nurses can offer advice on a wide range of health issues. You can also advocate for public health issues at your kids' school and in other settings. Doing so will educate those you help and those nearby that nurses have health expertise.

Nurses can also advocate for public health. Consider working for health financing reform, more school nurses, or food safety. Or work to improve the environment, reduce greenhouse gases, or find alternative sources of energy. You might even signal your personal virtue by conserving energy. Or help to address preventable global diseases. Nurses who fight for global health send the message that they believe in their profession, that they fight for their patients' needs whether they are at or away from the bedside. We're not saying you have to run for Congress or Parliament or something — though that might not be a bad idea, because we do need more nurses in power.

## Educate Physicians and Medical Students

Nurses already teach physicians a great deal about health care in clinical settings, but they could do more to tell them about nursing. In addition to nursing out loud, nurses might reach out to their local medical schools to emulate the Dartmouth shadowing program discussed in chapter 10. Nurses also might consider what Texas nurse practitioner Margaret Helminiak does: "When my physician colleague calls for a nurse but really means a medical assistant, I go into the room and tell her, 'You called for a nurse. I am the only nurse here. Everyone else is a medical assistant.'"

## Equal Rights for Equal Work

Address physicians as they address you. If they call you by your given name, call them by their given names. If a physician asks to be called "Dr. Jones," ask that the physician call you "Nurse Smith." If only senior physicians receive an honorific, ensure that senior nurses are treated the same way. This makes it clear to all — including the media — that physicians are not your masters or betters. You are colleagues, each deserving of respect.

## Tell Patients What Your Role Is

Nurses often have difficulty acting as the patient advocates they have been trained to be, especially when that role brings them into conflict with physicians. We propose a basic statement that nurses might consider making available to their patients and colleagues. The statement might go something like this:

---

### I AM YOUR REGISTERED NURSE

During your stay here, it is my duty to protect you from all harm. That means any harm from your illness and its symptoms, from external forces including the care environment, and from other people. As an autonomous health professional who reports only to senior nurses, it is my job to protect you from poor or misguided health care from any source. I am your advocate. I vow to do my best to protect you as if you were a member of my family.

---

# EDUCATING THE MEDIA ABOUT NURSING

Once you have embraced your own power to create change and considered what you can do every day to improve the image of nursing, please take a look at what the media is saying about your profession. Does it reflect the stereotypes we have discussed in this book? Next we discuss some ideas we have found useful in helping the media improve.

## Develop Media Expertise and Get Coverage for Nursing

We urge nurses to accept responsibility for the central role they play in health care, even when there are problems. Nurses must stand up and be someone when the media is around — not simply defer to physicians, or slink into corners, as some nurses do.

1) **Read *From Silence to Voice*.** The excellent book by Bernice Buresh and Suzanne Gordon is *the* how-to manual for nurses seeking to relate to the media. Every nurse should read it.

2) **Observe experts on major media outlets.** Every day, highly skilled experts in various fields present their views on television and radio networks, and in print media articles. Consider how these experts relate to journalists, how they present their basic positions and respond to questions. Consider how well prepared they are. Then practice presenting your points and responding to possible questions.

3) **Study examples of good coverage of nursing.** Many press items have effectively highlighted nursing practice or research. In October 2008, the *New York Times* published a report about the research of Kristine Williams and colleagues at the University of Kansas, who found that use of "elderspeak" ("dear," "sweetie," "honey") causes patients to become aggressive and sends a message of incompetence, which starts them on a downward health trajectory. In March 2006 the *Mainichi Daily News* published a piece about research by Japanese nurses who showed that when patients listened to relaxing *enka* music during cardiac catheterizations, it lowered their blood pressure by forty-four points — thereby decreasing the risk of potentially lethal punctures to their heart vessels. And in February 2004 the Associated Press covered research led by nurse Cheryl Cmiel, who significantly lowered the noise level on her Mayo Clinic unit, allowing patients to rest better.

4) **Make it a priority to help media creators understand nursing when they ask.** When the media contacts us, we put everything else aside and talk for as long as they wish. We follow up immedi-

ately by sending documents or other resources to supplement the information we provided and answer any additional questions the media may have. In addition to providing input on stories about nursing in the media, we have been quoted in pieces discussing the nursing shortage, nursing uniforms, Magnet status, men in nursing, sexual abuse in nursing, and other topics. And we refer the media to other nurses with expertise. Please register in our expert database at www.nursingadvocacy.org/nurse_expert, and when appropriate, we will refer the media to you.

5) **Respond promptly.** The media moves quickly and media opportunities are usually fleeting. We once had a great television opportunity lined up for the director of a state nursing association, but she "had a meeting" that afternoon and couldn't do it. The issue was controversial, but this director could have used the chance to present her perspective and let viewers know that nursing leaders are responsive health professionals with opinions about public policy issues.

6) **Establish relationships with local media and persuade them to cover nursing.** Invite your local media people to lunch or coffee, and tell them about the diverse work of nurses. Set up a luncheon or roundtable at which local nursing leaders talk to the media about their innovative practices or research. Invite the media to nursing meetings and seminars. Nurse researchers should consider the last step in their publication process to be coverage in the lay media. Send the media your research and tell them why their readers would find it compelling. Nursing journal editors should seek coverage from mainstream health journalists. Or establish a Be a Nurse for a Day program so the media can follow nurses at work.

7) **Nurses did that!** Tell your best stories, but make sure the role of nurses is clear. The media needs to learn more about the dramatic work of nurses. The Center has a story idea database on its website, and we encourage nurses to submit their most dramatic stories — good and bad. Too often we hear that important care just "happened" (as if the hospital walls did it) or that "we" did it — both of which obscure the fact that *nurses* did it.

8) **Consider formal training.** If you will be appearing before the media with any frequency, we recommend in-person media training. Find more information at nursingadvocacy.org/action/media_training.html.

9) **Be nurse-identified.** Sometimes nurse experts appear in the media, but the piece simply identifies them as a PhD or as "Dr. Bivens" — without mentioning that the expert is a nurse. This leads the public to credit physicians or other non-nurses for this nurse's expertise or work. If forced to choose between RN and PhD identifiers, we urge nurses to choose the RN. As *Nursing Spectrum* editor Pam Meredith wrote in a 2002 editorial, "Pick up that RN flag and wave it."

10) **Don't let HIPAA paralyze you.** The HIPAA (Health Insurance Portability and Accountability Act) is designed to keep patient information confidential.[4] *It does not forbid nurses to speak about their work.* Overreacting to HIPAA can mean that nursing will be cut out of the media picture. One Johns Hopkins media professional involved with the 2008 ABC documentary *Hopkins* told us that the hospital used a standard release form to comply with HIPAA. He said that 95 percent of patients readily consented, in a process that sometimes took as little as twenty seconds. The

hospital also put the television crew that filmed *Hopkins* through the hospital's standard HIPAA training program, so they could get their own consents. And of course, even if nurses do not get release forms signed, they can still talk to the media about their work and patient care, as long as they disclose no information that identifies any specific patient.

## Catch the Media Being Good

Although we spend significant time trying to persuade the media to do a better job, we also try to provide as much positive reinforcement as we can. When we do see an accurate, enlightening depiction of nursing, we try to thank those responsible, even if only in a short email. Every nurse should consider doing the same.

A more formal way of reinforcing good portrayals of nursing is through the Center's annual Golden Lamp Awards. Each year since 2003, the Center has issued a list of the best and worst media portrayals of nursing it has seen in the previous year, along with some special awards for best efforts to improve. Naturally, most people like to be recognized for good work. When Tim Green, editor of the poetry magazine *Rattle*, began to prepare a special nursing issue, he asked for our guidance. He asked how he could make the issue worthy of one of our "ten best media depictions of the year" awards. He listened carefully to our views, though we played no role in his editorial choices. The issue's nurse-penned poetry was powerful, insightful, and devoid of stereotypes — and it did win a Golden Lamp for one of the best portrayals of 2007.

# Different Ways to Persuade the Media to Reconsider Products

The Center has spent significant time asking media creators to reconsider their products, from Hollywood shows to print advertising. In some cases, we have persuaded media creators to address our concerns with relatively little effort. Other campaigns have required major efforts, including thousands of letters and global media coverage. Here are some ways to reach media creators in different situations.

## PHONE CALLS

Sometimes the only tool required to affect media content is your telephone. In nearly all the Center's campaigns to improve poor portrayals of nursing, we first call media makers. Constellation Brands launched a multimedia naughty nurse ad campaign for Hydra vodka water in 2006. We called the vice president of corporate communications, who quickly decided to remove the nurse elements from the campaign. And when Bloomingdale's ran a radio ad in November 2007 featuring a "nurse" seducing a "physician" with a cashmere sweater, we called the company's senior VP of public relations, who quickly asked for something in writing, presumably to forward to colleagues. We sent an email in about half an hour. Two hours later, after the close of business on a Friday, Bloomingdale's told us that it had begun calling radio stations to prevent the ad from running over that busy holiday season shopping weekend. Of course, phone calls alone are not always enough. In those situations, we move to letters or letter-writing campaigns.

## LETTERS AND EMAILS

Sometimes it just takes one email to make a difference. In September 2006 we asked ALR Technologies to change the informal name of its

ALRT500 home health management device from Electronic Nurse to a name that did not suggest that the machine could replace a real nurse. In an email, we explained that the device does not make professional judgments and take skilled actions based on years of college-level science education, as nurses do. The company soon apologized and removed the nickname.

## LETTER-WRITING CAMPAIGNS

When the above efforts fail, it's usually time to turn up the heat. Letter-writing campaigns have been pivotal in many of our efforts to improve media on nursing. Sometimes a few letters are enough to get some result. When the quiz show *Jeopardy!* wrongly implied in 2004 that nurse practitioners treat only "minor ailments," a handful of letters were enough to persuade the producers to place a question on the show designed to improve understanding of nursing.

Some advertisers require more than a few letters. When Skechers launched its global ad campaign featuring Christina Aguilera as a dominatrix naughty nurse in 2005, the company was unresponsive to our calls. However, after our supporters sent three thousand emails over two weeks, Skechers removed the ads. In August 2008 the Registered Nurses Association of Ontario (RNAO) sent a letter asking Canada's Neilson Dairy to end use of naughty nurse models in ads and at a related extreme sports tour. RNAO's one letter did not move the company, but more than a thousand letters from RNAO supporters did. A week later the company apologized and promised to remove the naughty nurse imagery.

## PRESS RELEASES

When we launched our campaign in 2006 to ask the Heart Attack Grill in Arizona to remove the nurse theme from its waitresses' sexy costumes, we started with phone calls to the restaurant's owner. These interactions proved too much for him. We moved to emails and a letter-writing campaign, but those were not effective either. Next we issued a press release to every print and broadcast media outlet in Arizona and to major media outside the state. A local television station picked it up, and the story quickly spread into broadcast and major print sources across the United States and the world. Not everyone agreed with our position, and so far we have still not persuaded the Grill to reconsider its use of the naughty nurse. But tens of millions of people heard our message about nursing stereotypes and were asked to consider how the images affect nursing.

## UNORTHODOX APPROACHES

There are many ways to get the media's attention. For instance, the Center's annual Golden Lamp Awards include awards for the "worst portrayal of nursing." In 2006 we sent a "worst portrayal" award to rock star Jack White of the White Stripes, along with our analysis of his 2005 song "The Nurse." We explained how his lyrics associated a "nurse" with romantic love, mothering, and housekeeping. In response, White sent Sandy a satirical "Metaphorical Ignorance Award." White evidently did not get that we were actually objecting to his use of *metaphor* to reinforce nursing stereotypes: we did not imagine that his song was saying real nurses rubbed salt in his physical wounds. But having gotten his attention, we issued a press release about our mock-award exchange and got coverage for our issues in the *Los Angeles Times*, *Salon*, and elsewhere.

If you have significant resources, your options expand. The California Nurses Association (CNA) has used a wide variety of creative tactics, some controversial, to get its messages out. In the mid-2000s, after California governor Arnold Schwarzenegger opposed implementation of nurse staffing legislation that CNA had fought to pass, the union protested at his every appearance and used various ads to tell the public about the dangers of high nurse-to-patient ratios. After CNA won its campaign for minimum ratios, it set its sights on universal health coverage. In May 2008 CNA ran an ad in the *Washington Post* referring to Vice President Cheney's excellent federal government health insurance: "If [Cheney] were anyone else, he'd probably be dead by now."[5] Not everyone applauded these tactics, but they drew attention to CNA's issues.

## Persuading Media Decision Makers in Direct Interactions

Let's say you want to affect what a specific media creator is telling the public about nursing right now. How would you do it? We have some suggestions.

### IDENTIFY AND REACH THE DECISION MAKER

Many corporations have customer service phone numbers, but those who staff them usually have little decision-making power, and they often seem to be trained to deflect concerns about their media rather than address them. We have found them receptive in only one instance, when the head of customer service at Coors worked with us to convince the company's Canadian division to discontinue naughty nurse advertising in late 2006.

When we reach the person who has the power to decide how a specific media product is made or shown to the public, that person will often listen and work with us. But identifying the decision maker is not always easy. That person's identity depends on the medium. For the news media, the person you want is usually the reporter or an editor. In commercial advertising, it's usually the vice president of marketing, consumer affairs, or corporate communications. In television, it is generally the executive producers. In film, it is usually the director and the writer.

In 2002, when we first tried to persuade the U.S. government to reconsider the name of its Take a Loved One health campaign, Sandy called the Department of Health and Human Services' Office of Minority Health (OMH) main telephone line. She was transferred to a low-level official. We got nowhere. In 2004 we tried again, and this time we found the decision maker — the director of the OMH — but could not reach him by phone. So we launched a letter-writing campaign, and over three hundred supporters sent him emails. The director's assistant then agreed to set up a call between the director and Sandy. In a constructive discussion, he vowed to explore a better name for the campaign, and it was later changed.

In 2006 CVS ran television ads suggesting that a pharmacist had transformed a patient's spouse into a "nurse" after a few hours of training in how to give medications. We called CVS and were transferred to about fifteen different people and subdivisions of CVS over the course of four or five days. Finally we reached the company's VP of customer service. He was very helpful in working with us to remove the nurse element of the ad.

In 2007, Seattle's Group Health launched ads for its "Ask the Doc" service that included the tag line "Nurse, hand me my laptop," suggesting that nurses are there to fetch things for physicians. Several nurses at Group Health lobbied the company's marketing people to remove the ad, but they were told they had failed to appreciate the ad's "humor." So the nurses lobbied the CEO. He pulled the ad.

Although assistants and receptionists do not have decision-making authority, it is vital that you treat them with respect. That is not just because it's the right thing to do, but also because assistants often control access. Although your goal will generally be to get to their bosses, to do that you will often want to treat the assistants as if they *were* the decision makers. If you persuade them that your concern has merit — or at least that you are serious and will not waste their boss's time — you have a better chance of getting past them, and maybe even of influencing their presentation to their bosses to favor your view.

In general, if you're getting nowhere with the person you're dealing with, don't hesitate to politely go over his or her head. Just keep contacting people until you find the person who can make the decision. Be persistent!

## BE PERSISTENT!

If there is one tactic in getting the media to listen that supersedes all other tactics, it is *relentless persistence*. Make it clear that you will not go away until the person you are dealing with fixes the media problem. It does not always work, but often it does.

In 2007 Cadbury Schweppes Canada ran television commercials featuring female nurses hopping into bed with male patients who chewed Dentyne Ice gum. We called to discuss the ad. The company's director of corporate communications in Canada was notably unreceptive to our concerns. ("We test marketed it and no one complained that it was offensive!") For over a week we had daily conversations that yielded no positive result. So we launched a letter-writing campaign. The Registered Nurses Association of Ontario joined us and launched its own letter-writing campaign. But even after a combined 1,500 letters from our two groups, the communications director would not budge. In the meantime Sandy found the work phone numbers of the top seven Cadbury Schweppes executives in the world and began calling them daily, connecting primarily with their voicemail. She left them lengthy, detailed messages about the complex role media undervaluation plays in the global nursing shortage. After a week, the CEO of Cadbury Schweppes called Sandy from London to discuss her concerns and to tell her he was pulling the ad.

Physician inventor Michael Treat told the *New York Times* in 2005 that his new surgical robot Penelope "should be able to do everything a nurse can." We called Treat and spoke for ninety minutes about nursing, robots, and the nursing shortage. Treat was very friendly and thoughtful, but he didn't really seem to understand our concerns until about seventy-five minutes into our conversation. We convinced him that robots could not replace nurses in part because they could not advocate for patients, for instance by preventing inebriated surgeons from operating. In the phone call, Treat promised to stop telling the media that his robot can replace OR nurses, and as far as we know he has kept that promise.

## STUDY THE MEDIA PRODUCT AND ANTICIPATE ARGUMENTS

When preparing to contact media creators, it is important to look closely at the media product. Are parts of it ironic? Is it actually criticizing a stereotype rather than endorsing it? Media creators are more likely to listen if you show that you understand their work but still have an issue with it. Likewise, if a counter-argument is almost certain to be made, it may make sense to address it up front. This tactic may lessen resistance, or at least show that you have thought carefully about the issue. For example, when dealing with naughty nurse imagery, you can count on being told that it's "just a joke," though "jokes" are one of the most common ways to spread harmful stereotypes. We try to convey that we get the joke, or would appreciate a joke that was not so tired. When we contacted Fox News Channel's *Redeye* about an April 2008 show celebrating the naughty nurse stereotype, we presented our analysis in a satirical letter pretending to praise the show for embracing the stereotype.

## PLAY GOOD COP/BAD COP

Advocates may confront choices about whether to focus more on the "inside track" (such as by offering gentle private suggestions that might move powerful media creators slightly in the right direction) or the "outside track" (such as by offering rigorous public analysis of the meaning and effects of specific media products, which makes collaboration with creators less likely). We have adopted different approaches in different contexts, though we are better known for the outside approach. Of course, not everyone has to approach things the same way. We've noted that nursing has no shortage of "inside track" adherents.

In some cases, a combination of these approaches may be effective. Since 2001 we have been asking *ER* to improve its portrayal of nursing. For some time in the early 2000s, it was rare for the minor nurse characters to appear on the show. In contrast to the many physician characters, the one major nurse character had little clinical role, and she spent most of her time engaged in romances with physicians or enduring family tragedies. We had a lengthy, cordial conference call with an *ER* producer and the show's "medical" adviser in late 2001, but it was pretty clear the show did not really feel it needed our advice on an ongoing basis. So we began sending the show our critical analyses of its episodes and urging our supporters to pressure it to improve, and we have done so ever since.[6] We understand that the show did not like these efforts, though a stronger major nurse character (Sam Taggart) was introduced in late 2003.

In March 2005 we urged advertisers to withhold their ads until *ER* improved. The next month, the senior vice president of global medical affairs for pharmaceutical giant Schering-Plough, physician Hans Vemer, responded to our campaign by asking the show to help address the nursing shortage by developing "stories that highlight accurate roles, responsibilities, skills and contributions of today's modern nursing profession."

Meanwhile, we understand that Sojourn Communications, a Hollywood-based communications company, played a key role in helping *ER* develop the Eve Peyton plotlines of late 2005, which addressed some of our concerns about nursing skill and autonomy; indeed, some scenes might easily have been crafted by the Center. Peyton's exit drew heavily on the battle-axe image, but on the whole the episodes were helpful.

Since then, *ER* has at times made a point of displaying nursing autonomy and skill. October 2008 episodes even indicated that Taggart was starting a nurse anesthetist program, breaking the show's tradition of having major nurse characters aspire to medical school when they pursue graduate studies. There has been little more about nursing leaders or managers, and the physician-centric show still falls well short of a good portrayal of nursing, but on the whole, it has made a modest improvement.

## MOVE FAST

It is often easier to get the attention of media figures if you're able to connect with them soon after a troubling portrayal appears. That's especially true of talk radio. In June 2007, when radio host Stephanie Miller and sidekick Jim Ward had some fun with naughty nurse stereotyping, the Center sent them an analysis, and they promptly read and mocked parts of it on the air. Within minutes, a supporter called Sandy and she called the show, which allowed her on the air to briefly explain her concerns.

In January 2006, on Sean Hannity's radio show, one caller asked a U.S. soldier who had been an inpatient at Walter Reed Army hospital whether there were any "hot nurses" there. The soldier reportedly replied that there were "a few pretty ones" but that most were "motherly." A supporter notified the Center, and Sandy called Hannity's office. Twenty minutes later, Hannity himself called us back, and we talked about nursing stereotypes for some time. Hannity made supportive comments about nurses on the air in the following days.

## USE THE MEDIA'S OWN PROCESS

Some media creators have procedures for challenging their conduct. For example, in 2007 Heineken began running Dos Equis ads in which "the most interesting man in the world" bench-pressed two young women in short white dresses and nurses' caps. Following the advice of a Heineken corporate relations officer, the Center appealed to an independent board that handles such matters for Heineken, using codes of marketing that Heineken follows. Among other things, we argued that the ad violated the Heineken International Commercial Communication Code, which required that ads "be prepared with due regard for our social responsibility" and that they not "impugn human dignity and integrity." The review board, which included former U.S. vice presidential candidate Geraldine Ferraro, agreed that the ad should be changed. Heineken digitally altered the women's clothing to remove the nurse element and proceeded to air that version.

## COLLABORATE

In various campaigns, we have collaborated with the American College of Nurse Midwives, the American Academy of Nurse Practitioners, the Registered Nurses Association of Ontario, and other groups. Collaboration has created larger responses than we could on our own and made our campaigns much more effective. It was certainly a factor in successfully challenging the U.S. government's Take a Loved One to the Doctor campaign and the Dentyne Ice ad. Sometimes we have been able to get help from companies outside the nursing community, as we did when Schering-Plough wrote to *ER*. And when Mattel released its Nurse Quacktitioner doll, we convinced Wal-Mart to sell the dolls back to Mattel, as a way of adding pressure on Mattel. Unfortunately, Mattel did not agree to the buy-back.

## SUGGEST ALTERNATIVES

Media creators may be receptive if you suggest a way they can achieve their goals without reinforcing nursing stereotypes. In 2005 Wal-Mart placed an ad in nursing journals featuring a "nurse" and the tag line "It doesn't take a brain surgeon to recognize a good deal on scrubs." We contacted Wal-Mart to object to the ad's suggestion that nurses aren't all that smart. The company not only agreed to change the ad copy, but also took us up on our offer to help.

Sometimes it can be helpful to propose a specific alternative course to the media, even if there is little chance the media creator will adopt it. After reading our analysis of a damaging January 2007 episode of *Grey's Anatomy*, nurse Mandy Mayling of Los Angeles wrote and sent the show an alternative script. The inventive script showed how the episode might have featured at least as much drama while accurately representing nursing.

## EXPECT RESISTANCE

Change can be scary. So changing the way people think is not easy or quick. Since the beginning, the Center has faced vigorous opposition from some media creators and many of their supporters. Naughty nurse fans can be especially committed, but Hollywood shows and pop musicians also enjoy a good deal of blind loyalty. Some wonder how we keep going in the face of this. But we recall Mahatma Gandhi, who described social change this way:

First they ignore you;
Then they laugh at you;
Then they attack you;
Then you win.

Nursing has been largely absent from serious discussions of health care in the media for decades. It's not exactly encouraging to be laughed at or attacked, but we believe these are steps up from being ignored. And in some cases these reactions have been a prelude to achieving our immediate goal of improving a given media product — and, we believe, our larger goal of changing the way people think about nursing.

## Organize Chapters of the Center

The Center has local chapters all over the world, but we are looking for nurses to start more. Chapters meet periodically and consider ways to encourage local media to improve its coverage of nursing. If nurses in every media market worked together to implement the ideas in this chapter, the media all over the world would change the way it treats nursing. Please visit www.nursingadvocacy.org/chapters to get involved.

# MESSAGE IN A BOTTLE: CREATE YOUR OWN MEDIA

Nurses know best what nursing is and what nurses do, so they should explain their work to the world directly. Some nurses have actually become media professionals, which we encourage. But you don't need to be a media professional to create compelling media: you can even use a blog to improve understanding. Depending on their interests, nurses might use written work; visual, performance, and tactile media; and video, broadcast, and film.

## Writing about Nursing

Writing has many benefits as a way to help others understand nursing. It allows for precise, detailed explanation that can be very helpful for a profession that needs to convey complex skills and thought processes.

### LETTERS TO THE EDITOR

Letters to the editor are a great place for anyone to start. Letters can be as short as one paragraph, and they are easier to get published than some other types of traditional print media. Letters are often used to persuade the media to do better, but they can influence the public in their own right. For example, a February 2006 issue of *Good Housekeeping* included an effective letter from nurse Berni Martin protesting a feature from a past issue that had included a health tip from an anonymous ED physician that readers should lie to triage nurses in order to be seen faster. Not all letters need to respond to specific reports; some discuss issues of the day. In May 2005 the *Wawatay News* in Ontario published a Nursing Week letter to the editor by Canadian federal health nurse Lyn Button of the Sioux Lookout Zone. The letter provided special insight into what nurses do for patients in remote rural communities. Don't be dissuaded if your first letter doesn't get printed. Be persistent!

## OP-EDS

We urge nurses to write op-eds (opinion-editorial pieces), which can make powerful arguments about a wide variety of nursing issues. In December 2005 the *Milwaukee Journal Sentinel* published Gina Dennik-Champion's persuasive op-ed supporting pending legislation to authorize medical marijuana use. That same month the Toronto *Globe and Mail* ran a moving op-ed by Calgary maternity nurse Raewyn Janota, who described the skilled, sensitive care she provided to a couple whose baby was stillborn. And the previous May the *Post and Courier* of Charleston, South Carolina, published an op-ed by nursing dean Gail Stuart, who argued that her state's severe nursing shortage threatens not only residents' health but the state's economic well-being. Getting op-eds published is generally harder than getting letters published, especially if you are trying for a major periodical or have a message that editors do not expect to hear. When we got our op-ed arguing for a Nobel Prize in nursing published in the *Baltimore Sun* in December 2006, it was the culmination of *three years* of work. We revised the draft many times and submitted it to many publications before we succeeded. So be tenacious, revise, seek advice, and keep pitching your message.

## FEATURE ARTICLES

Nurses don't need to depend on reporters to cover them, because they can write about their own work! One common way to do that is through features, which describe interesting events or ideas that are not breaking news. These are often written in the first person, as many of the *New York Times* "Cases" items are, including oncology nurse Theresa Brown's September 2008 piece about the death of one of her patients. Another example is nurse John Blanton's excellent April 2007 *Wall Street Journal* article "Care and Chaos on the Night Nursing Shift" about his post-9/11 journey from *WSJ* editor to burn ICU nurse and back again. And nurse Sallie Tisdale's *Salon* piece of that same month, "The Beautiful Hospital," explained how prime-time Hollywood shows fail to convey what really goes on in hospitals like hers.

## NON-FICTION BOOKS

Many nurses have written non-fiction books to explain their nursing experience or help people with their expertise. Writing and publishing a book can be a challenge, but books can have a lasting impact. Nurse Echo Heron is well known for dramatic non-fiction books about her work and that of her colleagues, starting with the best-selling *Intensive Care: The Story of a Nurse* (1988). Nurse Pat Carroll's *What Nurses Know and Doctors Don't Have Time to Tell You* (2004) effectively explained important health principles to the lay public, though it was marred by a title that managed to both celebrate and denigrate nurses. In 2005 nurse Claire Bertschinger published *Moving Mountains* about her work caring for children in the 1980s Ethiopian famine — work that reportedly inspired the 1985 Live Aid benefit. Nurses Gloria Mayer and Ann Kuklierus have written three influential "plain talk" books for the public, including 1999's *What to Do When Your Child Gets Sick*, which is sent to the parents of every newborn California child courtesy of the state.[7] And nurse Cheryl Dellasega, an expert in relational aggression, writes books to help women and girls improve their relationships, including *Forced to Be Family* (2007) and *Surviving Ophelia* (2001).

## NOVELS

Novels can be a very powerful way to convey the nursing experience. The highest-profile novelist nurse is probably Echo Heron, who has written several hospital thrillers, including *Fatal Diagnosis* (2000) and *Mercy* (1992). Nurse Richard Ferri's *Confessions of a Male Nurse* (2006) was a funny account of a gay man in nursing, though we were uneasy with the way it presented the main character's love affair with a physician, which seemed to suggest that medicine had far greater value than nursing. Other nurses have written novels, but few prominent ones seem to focus on nursing. The world is waiting for yours!

## OTHER LITERATURE AND STORYTELLING

Nurses participate in compelling dramas every day: write about them! There are many print avenues besides novels for nurses who want to tell people something about nursing in a creative way. The poetry magazine *Rattle*'s special issue on nursing included many impressive nurse poets who explored the health care experience from a nurse's perspective. Nurses could tell the reading public something of what they do through short fiction, which is published in a variety of magazines. Nurses could even do so through comics. Garry Trudeau's 2004 *Doonesbury* strips about nurses caring for a wounded Iraq war veteran showed that comics could be helpful. Satirical pieces can also convey something of the nursing experience. In 2005 we issued an April Fool's Day press release about a groundbreaking study published in the *Journal of the American Medical Association* that had made the discovery that nurses are skilled, autonomous professionals who do vital work to improve public health. We included fake reaction from a variety of prominent media sources who professed shock. The "study" — which we invented — was entitled "Who Knew?"

## KIDS' LITERATURE

A compelling series of children's books about modern nursing could be very effective, especially since many children's books suggest that medicine is the really desirable health care career — particularly for ambitious girls. We need books to highlight nursing for toddlers, preschoolers, elementary kids, tweens, and teens. One series of novels that inspired many children to become nurses was the *Cherry Ames* series, originally published from 1943 to 1968. Springer Publishing reissued the series in 2005–2007, but the gender and nurse-physician relations are antiquated and unlikely to impress today's young readers. Nurse Serita Stevens wrote *Charlie London, RN* in 2004 to try to update the Cherry Ames series. The main nurse character was bright and positive, but we found that her reverence for physicians undermined the message about nursing. We need works that show nursing is as valuable and challenging as medicine. Of course, J. K. Rowling's Harry Potter books do include the very minor character Nurse Pomfrey, who is skilled at healing in a supernatural setting. But we need nurses to put nursing center stage. Maybe Harry Potter could become a flight nurse; that broom would be pretty quick to accident scenes!

## THE INTERNET: WEBSITES, BLOGS, AND DISCUSSION BOARDS

In 2008 the Internet was estimated to have about 1.5 billion users worldwide, including most of the public in the developed world. Virtually all the written media forms discussed above are now available online. The Internet is the main way the Center interacts with the media and the public. The Infobahn offers countless communication avenues that might help nurses tell the public what they do. We discuss a few next.

Many nursing discussion boards and weblogs (blogs) are available to all Internet users. So they are obviously important ways to spread information to the public about who nurses are and what they do. Some do a good job of exploring current nursing issues. But some popular nursing discussion boards do not always convey to members of the public who stumble upon them that nurses are well-educated professionals. Of course, these are places nurses go to vent and discuss their very real work difficulties. But we urge nurses to consider if their posts would inspire decision makers to give nursing the resources it needs.

Websites have become an essential communication tool. Some nurse-created sites try to give the public information about what nursing is, including the Center's www.nursingadvocacy.org. Sandy also played a substantial role in creating the information about nursing on Johnson & Johnson's www.discovernursing.com.

Nurses should consider creating or enhancing websites to explain nursing, including the sites of their employers and professional groups. Websites are now the public face of an organization. Use them to explain nursing at your institution to the public. Nursing schools often do profile their faculty, letting the public know about professors' credentials and interests. But try finding anything about a specific nurse on a hospital website. We have not seen one that highlights nursing care or the people who deliver it in any detail, much less the detail devoted to physicians, even though hospitals exist mainly to provide nursing care.

Make sure that your institution's website conveys the key role nurses play. To develop a website, ask media relations professionals for help. You might profile each nursing service and individual nurses. The public should be able to learn who is doing the nursing, including the nurses' credentials. Include headshots and contact information for each nurse. What innovations have your nurses played a role in? How is the institution working to improve nursing care? Consider including photos, audio, and video, which nurses might use to discuss their work and its importance to patients. Be sure it is easy to get to the nursing material from the site's main page.

Many people look for health information on the Internet. Nurses can use websites to educate their patients or communities about health, and in doing so, about nursing expertise. In today's managed care environment, many patients get home after a hospital visit with little idea how to manage their conditions. They may not understand how to use their crutches, monitor their wounds, test their blood sugar levels, exercise, or avoid foods that put them at risk. Even when nurses do manage to give patients this information, patients may forget or simply be overwhelmed. The Internet can be a great way to fill this need, and perhaps prevent future hospitalizations. And consider becoming certified by Health on the Net, a foundation that guides consumers to reliable health websites.[8]

## Visual, Performance, and Tactile Media

Nurses can also use many exciting types of media to *show* the world what they do and why it matters. Memorials, exhibits, and other media can help shape the public's view of nursing and its history. We have already proposed an international museum of modern nursing, which nurses should play the key role in establishing.

Some nurses have taken the lead in developing effective visual displays. When nurse Diane Carlson Evans realized that the two U.S. Vietnam war memorials in Washington, DC failed to include nurses' contributions, she spent nine years lobbying legislators and the public. The result was the U.S. Vietnam Women's Memorial, a statue of three nurses and a patient involved in a hopeful rescue operation.

In 2003 nurses at the University of Pennsylvania played a key role in organizing the Philadelphia Fabric Workshop and Museum's exhibit RN: The Past, Present and Future of the Nurses' Uniform. This exhibit was the source of the RN patches discussed earlier, which enable nurses to identify themselves to patients and colleagues.

The excellent *American Journal of Nursing* has twice sponsored Faces of Caring: Nurses at Work, a contest designed to capture the best photographs of nurses. Some winning photos were among the best still images of nurses we have seen. Only some of the photos were taken by nurses themselves; we encourage more nurses to take photographs of their colleagues at work.

Nurses who have made their mark in pop music include Naomi Judd, and John Darnielle of the Mountain Goats. But we are not aware that many nurses have created music that addresses nursing directly, as Sonic Youth's *Sonic Nurse* (2004) did. Nurses should consider it.

Plays and other spoken performances are compelling media that more nurses should consider. *Nurse!* was a one-woman off-Broadway play sponsored by the New York State Nurses Association. Based on actual nurses' strikes, the 2003 play's characters faced the dilemma of working mandatory overtime or losing their jobs. Some nurses also do comedy performances that convey some of the nursing experience. Hawaii's Hob Osterlund has a comic alter ego called Ivy Push, who hosts the "Chuckle Channel," which aims to improve patient health through laughter. NICU nurse Greg Williams does nurse-themed stand-up comedy in Atlanta, Georgia.

Stamps and other collectible items can help nursing. The U.S. Postal Service honored nurse midwifery pioneer Mary Breckinridge with a commemorative stamp in 1999. In October 2008 the American College of Nurse-Midwives worked with the post office to create a stamp series about nurse midwife care, which can be seen at www.photostamps.com/acnm. We encourage nurses to consider lobbying the postal service for more stamps to help educate the public about nursing.

Toys and games can also teach about nursing. When our son was four, he told us that boys couldn't be nurses. So we gave him the Archie McPhee "Male Nurse Action Figure," and he changed his mind. Nurses should also consider designing board games and video games to educate kids about nursing. Nurses might design a counterpart to Milton Bradley's legendary Operation game. How about Post-Operation, in which "nurse" players prevent infections, cardiovascular collapse, and other complications by observing shifting patient conditions and responding with quick actions? Or a new multiplayer version of video game Grand Theft Auto in which nurse players have to teach the gravely wounded criminal player how to do his complex self-care and embrace a healthy lifestyle? Cool!

## Video, Broadcast, and Film

The broadcast media (television and radio) and film are traditionally harder for creators to make use of than some other media. But with the explosion of information technology in recent decades, nurses can now create and post on the Internet helpful video and audio with far less effort.

### VIDEO

Videos can now be created and made available to the world with minimal equipment and technical expertise. Web videos posted on YouTube are extremely popular, especially among young people we need to recruit to nursing. Nurse-created Web works could range from short recruiting videos to longer discussions of the profession or general health topics, such as nurse Barbara Ficarra's online video series *Nurses in Motion* on ScribeMedia.org. In particular, children's videos (like children's books) tend to present medicine as the only career really worth pursuing in health care, and countering that myth might be especially helpful.

Nurses have already created some compelling Web video. One of the best short works we've seen is the irreverent 2004 rap video created by ED nurse Craig Barton at the University of Alabama. In 2004 Liz Dubelman posted a gripping, innovative "VidLit" (literature-based flash animation) based on nurse Veneta Masson's poem "The Arithmetic of Nurses," about a home care nurse's work with a "sick old man." Masson's matter-of-fact text charted the human spirit straining to break through physical decay and social neglect. And in late 2006 students at Binghamton University's nursing school posted a recruiting video called "We're Bringing Nursing Back," which was based on Justin Timberlake's electrofunk hit "SexyBack." In the video, the students danced to the backing track but altered the song's lyrics to extol the virtues of nursing. The video had its problems — for one, it failed to get across that nurses use advanced skills to save lives — but the students deserve credit for an audacious effort to attract career seekers.

## RADIO

Radio remains a very effective way to communicate, especially now that even a small station's programming can be delivered globally on the Web. Almost every community has radio stations, and every station needs a health show hosted by nurses. The gold standard of nurse-hosted radio shows is *HealthStyles*, hosted by Diana Mason and Barbara Glickstein, on WBAI in New York. It features nurses as experts on nearly every show, and when physicians are on, the hosts treat them as colleagues, not gods. Another nurse-hosted radio show is Barbara Ficarra's weekly *Health in 30* on New York's WRCR. Unfortunately, the show usually consults physicians for general health issues even when nurses would be just as helpful.

## TELEVISION AND FILM

Television and film are very influential. Recently there have been a few relatively helpful films and television shows, such as Mike Nichols's *Angels in America* and documentaries including the *Nursing Diaries* installment by Richard Kahn and Helen Holt's *Nurses*. Nurses were instrumental in the creation of some of these media. However, as we have explained, the most influential products — such as Hollywood television dramas — remain very troubling. Nurses with the resources and skills should consider taking a more active role in producing, writing, and advising on these media.

Some nurses are leading the way. Nurse practitioner Ruth Tanyi produced, directed, and hosted a television series about diabetes called *Bad Sugar*, broadcast on California's KHIZ-TV in 2006 and 2007. Tanyi took a holistic look at the epidemic and explained how to avoid or at least control the disease by focusing on lifestyle, including diet, rest, and exercise. There will likely be a demand for more of this type of educational programming as the population ages and more people take an interest in long-term health management. Nurses are well placed to convey the needed health expertise — and in the process, to show the public that they *are* health experts.

Nurses should also consider developing ideas and writing scripts for a wide variety of entertainment programming, from reality shows to adult and teen dramas to children's programs like *Blue's Clues* and *Handy Manny*. It would be helpful if such scripts included just one nurse character who displayed some level of autonomy and skill, as physician characters do. A few years ago we tried to show that a nurse-focused television drama could be done by writing a sample script, which is available on the Center's website at www.nursingadvocacy.org/create/human.html.

As we conclude this book in late 2008, there are a few glimmers of light on the horizon for television featuring nurses, though the extent of nurse involvement in the programs varies. It appears that Showtime's comedy *Nurse Jackie* will air in early 2009. TNT is reportedly preparing a drama called *Time Heals* about the director of nursing at a North Carolina hospital. Nurse Serita Stevens is working with Canadian Television to develop a pilot based on her book *Forensic Nurse*. A successful Hollywood producer recently contacted the Center for extensive advice about a drama she is pitching, and we are also consulting on a possible reality show about nurses. The potential influence of these efforts is unclear, but all are worth pursuing to show the public what nurses really do.

## IT'S UP TO US

When the public does not understand the value of what nurses do — when nurses seem to have written in invisible ink — nursing cannot get the respect and resources it needs, and people suffer and die. We can all help resolve this global public health crisis, especially by improving the media portrayals that play such a critical role. We can change things. We live in a world in which women and racial minorities can hold the highest public offices, a reality that would have shocked many people a hundred years ago. The change is the result of relentless persistence and hard work: as Albert Camus said, tasks are called "superhuman" when they take a long time to complete, that is all.

Together we can create a world that allocates the resources nursing needs to save the lives of millions, and in which parents encourage bright children of both genders to become nurses. We can create a world that understands what one nurse's aunt learned, in a story the nurse later told us:

> I remember my aunt, who was an author, telling me I "could do better than that," and be a physician or a writer, as I so love to write. She would often say, "Why be just a nurse? You are wasting yourself in such a lowly profession." But you know, when she was dying of breast cancer, I stayed at her house with her (she lived alone) for her last two weeks. I felt honored to be able to be there as her favorite niece…and as her nurse. The night before she died she said this: "What would I do without you? Thank God you are a nurse." This was the last thing she said to me.

# ACKNOWLEDGMENTS

Many people deserve credit for helping us reach this point.

We owe a great deal to others who have explored how the media presents nursing, particularly journalists Suzanne Gordon and Bernice Buresh, and scholars Beatrice Kalisch and Philip Kalisch. We salute the nursing leaders who have inspired us and given us tireless support over the years, especially Claire Fagin, Diana Mason, and Linda Pugh. We thank the Center for Nursing Advocacy, for which much of the analysis adapted for this book was created. And we appreciate the vital contributions of Center supporters and staff, especially Joan Summers, Jack Summers, Lucille McCarthy, Hope Keller, Kelly Chew, and Sania Tildon.

Cole Summers, Simone Summers, and Harry F. Jacobs graciously tolerated our absences and the stresses associated with the writing of this book.

Our editor Shannon Berning provided insights and understanding, and everyone at Kaplan Publishing helped us complete this project under difficult circumstances.

Finally, we thank everyone who has helped us tell the public what nurses really do.

# ENDNOTES

## CHAPTER 1: Who Are Nurses and Where Have They Gone?

1 Center for Nursing Advocacy, "Q: Are You Sure Nurses Are Autonomous? Based on What I've Seen, It Sure Looks Like Physicians Are Calling the Shots," www.nursingadvocacy.org/faq/autonomy.html.

2 U.S. Department of Health and Human Services, Health Resources Services Administration, "The Registered Nurse Population: Findings from the 2004 National Sample Survey of Registered Nurses," http://bhpr.hrsa .gov/healthworkforce/rnsurvey04/ (accessed May 31, 2008).

3 Center for Nursing Advocacy, "Enemy of the People," www.nursingadvocacy .org/news/2005jun/22_dr_death.html.

4 Center for Nursing Advocacy, "Infirmières Sans Frontières," www.nursing advocacy.org/news/2006/dec/msf.html.

5 Bernice Buresh and Suzanne Gordon, *From Silence to Voice*, 2nd ed. (Ithaca: Cornell University Press, 2006); Suzanne Gordon, *Nursing Against the Odds: How Health Care Cost-Cutting, Media Stereotypes, and Medical Hubris Undermine Nursing and Patient Care* (Ithaca: Cornell University Press, 2005).

6 American Assembly of Men in Nursing, "The Story of Men in American Nursing," www.geocities.com/Athens/Forum/6011/sld024.htm, and www .geocities.com/Athens/Forum/6011/sld026.htm (accessed June 1, 2008).

7 Gina Castlenovo, "Mary Breckinridge," Center for Nursing Advocacy, www.nursingadvocacy.org/press/pioneers/breckinridge.html.

8 Foundation of New York State Nurses, Inc., Bellevue Alumnae Center for Nursing History, "Loeb Center for Nursing and Rehabilitation Records," http://foundationnysnurses.org/collections/loebfa.htm (accessed June 1, 2008).

9 Cynthia Adams, "Florence Wald: Pioneer in Hospice Care," Center for Nursing Advocacy, www.nursingadvocacy.org/press/pioneers/florence_wald.html.

10 Johns Hopkins University School of Nursing, "Jacquelyn Campbell, PhD, RN, FAAN," www.son.jhmi.edu/aboutus/directory/faculty/jcampbell.aspx (accessed June 1, 2008).

11 Johns Hopkins University School of Nursing, "Gayle Page, DNSc, RN, FAAN," www.son.jhmi.edu/aboutus/directory/faculty/gpage.aspx (accessed October 18, 2008).

12 University of Texas, "What Is Health Informatics?" www.shis.uth.tmc.edu/about-us/what-is-health-informatics (accessed June 1, 2008).

13 International Association of Forensic Nurses, "What Is Forensic Nursing?" www.forensicnurse.org/displaycommon.cfm?an=1&subarticlenbr=137 (accessed November 29, 2008).

14 Florence Nightingale International Foundation, "The International Achievement Award: Susie Kim (2001), RN DNSc, FAAN," www.fnif.org/awards.htm#SK (accessed October 18, 2008).

15 Geoffrey Cowley, "The Life of a Virus Hunter," *Newsweek,* May 15, 2006, www.stephenlewisfoundation.org/news_item.cfm?news=958&year=2006 (accessed October 18, 2008).

16 Dianne Hales, "The Quiet Heroes," *Parade,* March 21, 2004, www.parade.com/articles/editions/2004/edition_03-21-2004/featured_0 (accessed October 18, 2008).

17 University of Pennsylvania School of Nursing, "Linda Aiken," www.nursing.upenn.edu/faculty/profile.asp?pid=107 (accessed June 1, 2008).

18 Florence Nightingale International Foundation, "Awards: Carol Etherington (2003), MSN, RN, FAAN," www.fnif.org/awards.htm#CE (accessed June 1, 2008).

19 Johns Hopkins University School of Nursing, "Jacquelyn Campbell, PhD, RN, FAAN," www.son.jhmi.edu/aboutus/directory/faculty/jcampbell.aspx (accessed June 1, 2008).

20 Phuong Ly, "A Labor Without End," *Washington Post,* May 27, 2007, W20, www.washingtonpost.com/wp-dyn/content/article/2007/05/23/AR2007052301294.html (accessed November 30, 2008).

21 American Hospital Association, "The 2007 State of America's Hospitals—Taking the Pulse," www.aha.org/aha/content/2007/PowerPoint/StateofHospitalsChartPack2007.ppt (accessed June 1, 2008).

22  Arlene Dohm and Lynn Shniper, "Occupational Employment: Employ-
    ment Outlook: 2006–16: Occupational Employment Projections to 2016,"
    U.S. Department of Labor, Bureau of Labor Statistics, *Monthly Labor
    Review* (November 2007): 112, www.bls.gov/opub/mlr/2007/11/art5full.pdf
    (accessed November 30, 2008). See also U.S. Department of Labor, Bureau
    of Labor Statistics, "Occupational Outlook Handbook, 2008-09 Edition,
    Registered Nurses," www.bls.gov/oco/ocos083.htm (accessed November 30,
    2008).

23  Peter Buerhaus, Douglas Staiger and David Auerbach, *The Future of the
    Nursing Workforce in the United States: Data, Trends and Implications* (Bos-
    ton: Jones and Bartlett Publishers, 2008). For more information see Amer-
    ican Association of Colleges of Nursing, "Nursing Shortage Resource,"
    www.aacn.nche.edu/media/shortageresource.htm (accessed June 1, 2008).

24  Center for Nursing Advocacy, "What Happens To Patients When Nurses
    Are Short-Staffed?" www.nursingadvocacy.org/faq/short-staffed.html.

25  Alan H. Rosenstein, "Nurse-Physician Relationships: Impact on Nurse
    Satisfaction and Retention," *American Journal of Nursing* 102, no. 6
    (June 2002): 26-34, www.nursingcenter.com/library/JournalArticle.asp?
    Article_ID=278949 (accessed November 30, 2008).

26  Center for Nursing Advocacy, "Q: What Is Physician Disruptive Behav-
    ior and Why Does it Exist?" www.nursingadvocacy.org/faq/disruptive_
    behavior.html.

27  Suzanne Gordon, John Buchanan and Tanya Bretherton, *Safety in Numbers*
    (Ithaca: Cornell University Press, 2008); Suzanne Gordon, *Nursing Against
    the Odds: How Health Care Cost-Cutting, Media Stereotypes, and Medical
    Hubris Undermine Nursing and Patient Care,* (Ithaca: Cornell University
    Press, 2005); Dana Beth Weinberg, *Code Green: Money-Driven Hospitals
    and the Dismantling of Nursing* (Ithaca: Cornell University Press, 2003).
    For more information see Center for Nursing Advocacy, "What Happens
    To Patients When Nurses Are Short-Staffed?" www.nursingadvocacy.org/
    faq/short-staffed.html.

28  Linda Aiken, Sean Clarke, Douglas Sloane, Julie Sochalski and Jeffrey
    Silber, "Hospital Nurse Staffing and Patient Mortality, Nurse Burnout,
    and Job Dissatisfaction," *Journal of the American Medical Association*
    288, no. 16 (October 23-30, 2002): 1987-93. For more information see
    www.nursingadvocacy.org/news/2002oct23_jama.html.

29  Paul Duke, "If ER Nurses Crash, Will Patients Follow?" *Newsweek,* February 2, 2004. For more information see www.nursingadvocacy.org/news/2004feb/02_newsweek.html.

30  Anonymous, "One Day in Critical Care: A Nurse's Story," *Reader's Digest,* October 2003. See also Center for Nursing Advocacy, "Reader's Digest: Burnt-out ICU Nurse 'Blows the Whistle,'" www.nursingadvocacy.org/news/20030ct_rd.html.

31  Center for Nursing Advocacy, "What Happens To Patients When Nurses Are Short-Staffed?" www.nursingadvocacy.org/faq/short-staffed.html.

32  Linda Aiken, Sean Clarke, Douglas Sloane, Julie Sochalski and Jeffrey Silber, "Hospital Nurse Staffing and Patient Mortality, Nurse Burnout, and Job Dissatisfaction," *Journal of the American Medical Association* 288, no. 16 (October 23-30, 2002): 1987-93. For more information see www.nursingadvocacy.org/news/20020ct23_jama.html.

33  Jack Needleman, Peter Buerhaus, Maureen Stewart, Katya Zelevinsky and Soeren Mattke, "Nurse Staffing In Hospitals: Is There A Business Case For Quality?" *Health Affairs* 25, no. 1 (2006): 204–11. For more information see Center for Nursing Advocacy, "No magic number," www.nursingadvocacy.org/news/2006/jan/21_abc.html.

34  International Council of Nurses, "The Global Shortage of Registered Nurses: An Overview of Issues and Actions," www.icn.ch/global/shortage.pdf (accessed November 30, 2008).

35  Mireille Kingma, "Nurses On the Move: A Global Overview," *Health Services Research* 42, no. 3 (March 20, 2007): 1281-98, www3.interscience.wiley.com/journal/117996596/abstract. See also Mireille Kingma, *Nurses on the Move: Migration and the Global Health Care Economy* (Ithaca: Cornell University Press, 2006). For more information see Center for Nursing Advocacy, "Q: How Is Nurse Migration Affecting Nurses and the Nursing Shortage?" www.nursingadvocacy.org/faq/migration.html.

36  California Nurses Association, "RN-to-Patient Ratios," www.calnurses.org/nursing-practice/ratios/ratios_index.html (accessed November 30, 2008); Massachusetts Nurses Association, "Safe Care Campaign," www.massnurses.org/safe_care/index.htm (accessed June 1, 2008); Brian Bandell, "Shortage of Nurses Putting Patients at Risk," MSNBC, www.msnbc.msn.com/id/4587667/ (accessed June 1, 2008) (Florida proposals).

37  American Association of Colleges of Nursing, "Nurse Reinvestment Act at a Glance," www.aacn.nche.edu/Media/NRAataglance.htm (accessed June 1, 2008).

38  Center for Nursing Advocacy, "Q: How Is Nurse Migration Affecting Nurses and the Nursing Shortage?" www.nursingadvocacy.org/faq/migration.html.

39  Dennis O'Brien, "Nurses To Go," *Baltimore Sun,* March 17, 2006, http://tinyurl.com/67vgbw (accessed November 30, 2008); Center for Nursing Advocacy, "Would You Like a Krabby Patty with That?" www.nursingadvocacy.org/news/2006/mar/17_balt_sun.html.

40  Center for Nursing Advocacy, "What Is Magnet Status and How's that Whole Thing Going?" www.nursingadvocacy.org/faq/magnet.html.

41  Center for Nursing Advocacy, "Touching the World," www.nursingadvocacy.org/media/commercials/jnj_2005.html; Center for Nursing Advocacy, "Baby We Were Born To Care," www.nursingadvocacy.org/media/commercials/jnj_2007.html.

42  Nurses for a Healthier Tomorrow, "Careers in Nursing Campaign," www.nursesource.org/campaign_newsCIN.html (accessed June 1, 2008).

43  American Association of Colleges of Nursing, "Nursing Faculty Shortage Fact Sheet," www.aacn.nche.edu/Media/backgrounders/facultyshortage.htm (accessed June 1, 2008).

44  National League for Nursing, "Key Findings of Nationwide NLN-Carnegie Foundation: Study of Nurse Educators Released," www.nln.org/newsreleases/carnegie_082907.htm (accessed October 18, 2008).

45  National Institutes of Health, "Summary of the FY 2009 President's Budget," http://tinyurl.com/27lkm3 (accessed May 31, 2008).

46  Peter Buerhaus, Douglas Staiger and David Auerbach, *The Future of the Nursing Workforce in the United States: Data, Trends and Implications* (Boston: Jones and Bartlett Publishers, 2008) www.jbpub.com/catalog/9780763756840/ (accessed November 30, 2008). For more information see American Association of Colleges of Nursing, "Nursing Shortage Resource," www.aacn.nche.edu/media/shortageresource.htm (accessed June 1, 2008).

47  Press Trust Of India, "India Running Short of Two Million Nurses," *The Hindu*, March 17, 2008, http://tinyurl.com/6zg6n2 (accessed December 2, 2008).

48  Carol Natukunda, "Uganda: Where Did All the Nurses Go?" *New Vision* (Kampala), March 17, 2008, http://allafrica.com/stories/200803171613.html (accessed June 1, 2008).

**CHAPTER 2:** How Nursing's Image Affects Your Health

1  Center for Nursing Advocacy, "Q: Nurses Are Just Wonderful, But You Really Can't Expect Hollywood To Focus on Them, Can You? After All, Popular Media Products Have To Be Dramatic and Exciting. Why Don't You Just Focus on Getting a Nursing Documentary on PBS or Basic Cable?" www.nursingadvocacy.org/faq/dramatic.html.

2  The University of Rochester School of Nursing, "Woodhull Study on Nursing and the Media: Health Care's Invisible Partner," Sigma Theta Tau International (1997), www.nursingsociety.org/Media/Pages/woodhall.aspx (accessed November 27, 2008); Bernice Buresh, Suzanne Gordon, and Nica Bell, "Who Counts in News Coverage of Health Care?" *Nursing Outlook* 39, no. 5 (September / October 1991): 204-8.

3  Beatrice J. Kalisch and Philip A. Kalisch, "Anatomy of the Image of the Nurse: Dissonant and Ideal Models," *American Nurses Association Publications* G-161 (1983): 3-23. See generally Center for Nursing Advocacy, "The Work of Beatrice Kalisch and Philip Kalisch on Nursing's Public Image and the Nursing Shortage," www.nursingadvocacy.org/research/lit/kalisch_kalisch.html.

4  Deborah Glik, "Health Communication in Popular Media Formats" (paper presented at the 131st annual meeting of the American Public Health Association, San Francisco, California, November 15–19, 2003), www.medscape.com/viewarticle/466709 (accessed November 27, 2008).

5  Joseph Turow and Rachel Gans, "As Seen on TV: Health Policy Issues in TV's Medical Dramas," Kaiser Family Foundation (2002), www.kff.org/entmedia/3231-index.cfm (accessed June 1, 2008).

6  Suzanne Gordon and Bernice Buresh, "Doc Hollywood," *The American Prospect,* May 20, 2001, www.prospect.org/cs/articles?article=doc_hollywood (accessed November 30, 2008).

7  Lisa Liddane, "Paging Dr. Nielsen: TV medical shows," *Orange County Register,* October 8, 2006. For more information see www.nursingadvocacy.org/faq/media_affects_thinking.html.

8  Carol Ann Campbell, "Nurses Urge TV Dramas: Get Real," *New Jersey Star-Ledger,* January 28, 2007. For more information see www.nursingadvocacy.org/news/2007/jan/28_star_ledger.html.

9  Allison Van Dusen, "Playing Doctor: Medical TV Isn't Always Right," *Forbes,* September 20, 2007, www.msnbc.msn.com/id/20895520/ (accessed December 2, 2008).

10 JWT Communications, "Memo to Nurses for a Healthier Tomorrow Coalition Members on a Focus Group Study of 1800 School Children in 10 US Cities," 2000, www.nursingadvocacy.org/research/lit/jwt_memo1 .html.

11 Kaiser Family Foundation, "Entertainment Education and Health in the United States" (2004), www.kff.org/entmedia/7047.cfm (accessed June 1, 2008); U.S. Centers for Disease Control and Prevention, "Porter Novelli Healthstyles Survey" (2000), www.cdc.gov/healthmarketing/ entertainment_education/2000Survey.htm (accessed June 1, 2008).

12 Susan E. Morgan, Tyler R. Harrison, Lisa Chewning, LaShara Davis and Mark DiCorcia, "Entertainment (Mis)Education: The Framing of Organ Donation in Entertainment Television," *Health Communication* 22, no. 2 (August 2007): 143-51, www.purdue.edu/dp/rche/donatelife/ Entertainment_miseducation.pdf (accessed June 1, 2008).

13 Susan Morgan, Tyler Harrison, Shawn Long, Walid Afifi, Michael Stephenson and Tom Reichert, "Family Discussions about Organ Donation: How the Media Influences Opinions about Donation Decisions," *Clinical Transplantation* 19, no. 5 (2005): 674-82, www.blackwell-synergy. com/doi/abs/10.1111/j.1399-0012.2005.00407.x (accessed June 1, 2008); Richard J. Crockett, Thomas Pruzinsky and John A. Persing, "The Influence of Plastic Surgery 'Reality TV' on Cosmetic Surgery Patient Expectations and Decision Making," *Plastic & Reconstructive Surgery* 120, no. 1 (July 2007): 316-24, http://tinyurl.com/6y97d3 (accessed November 30, 2008). See Kathleen Doheny, "Cosmetic Surgery TV Shows Get Viewers Pondering," *HealthDay,* August 9, 2007, http://abcnews.go.com/Health/ Healthday/story?id=4508234 (accessed December 1, 2008).

14 Victoria Rideout, "Television as a Health Educator: A Case Study of *Grey's Anatomy*," Kaiser Family Foundation (September 16, 2008), www.kff.org/ entmedia/7803.cfm (accessed November 28, 2008).

15 Michael M. O'Connor, "The Role of the Television Drama *ER* in Medical Student Life: Entertainment or Socialization?" *Journal of the American Medical Association* 280, no. 9 (September 2, 1998): 854-55, http://jama .ama-assn.org/cgi/content/full/280/9/854 (accessed November 30, 2008).

16 Kaiser Family Foundation, "Entertainment Education and Health in the United States" (2004), http://tinyurl.com/2h57qq (accessed June 1, 2008); Mollyann Brodie, Ursula Foehr, Vicky Rideout, Neal Baer, Carolyn Miller, Rebecca Flournoy and Drew Altman, "Communicating Health Information through the Entertainment Media," *Health Affairs* 20, no. 1 (January/

February 2001): 192-9, http://content.healthaffairs.org/cgi/reprint/20/1/192 (accessed June 1, 2008); Kaiser Family Foundation, "The Impact of TV's Health Content: A Case Study of ER Viewers" (2002), www.kff.org/entmedia/3230-index.cfm (accessed June 1, 2008).

17  Thomas Valente, Sheila Murphy, Grace Huang, Jodi Gusek, Jennie Greene and Vicki Beck, "Evaluating a Minor Storyline on ER about Teen Obesity, Hypertension, and 5 A Day," Journal of Health Communication 12, no. 6 (September 2007): 551-66, www.comminit.com/es/node/70268 (accessed June 1, 2008).

18  Harvard School of Public Health, "After 'ER' Smallpox Episode, Fewer 'ER' Viewers Report They Would Go to Emergency Room If They Had Symptoms of the Disease" (June 13, 2002 press release), www.hsph .harvard.edu/news/press-releases/archives/2002-releases/press06132002 .html (accessed June 1, 2008).

19  RAND Health, "Entertainment TV Can Help Teach Teens Responsible Sex Messages," www.rand.org/health/healthpubs/friends.html (accessed June 1, 2008), citing Rebecca Collins, Marc Elliott, Sandra Berry, David Kanouse and Sarah Hunter, "Entertainment Television as a Healthy Sex Educator: The Impact of Condom Efficacy Information in an Episode of Friends," Pediatrics 112, no. 5 (November 2003): 1115-21, http://pediatrics.aappublications.org/cgi/content/abstract/112/5/1115 (accessed June 1, 2008).

20  Kaiser Family Foundation, "Entertainment Education and Health in the United States" (2004), www.kff.org/entmedia/7047.cfm, citing U.S. Centers for Disease Control and Prevention, "Soap Opera Viewers and Health Information: 1999 Healthstyles Survey," http://tinyurl.com/5g2gkq (accessed June 1, 2008).

21  A. O'Leary, M. Kennedy, V. Beck, P. Simpson and K. Pollard, "Increases in Calls to the CDC's National STD and AIDS Hotline Following AIDS-Related Episodes in a Soap Opera," Journal of Communication 54, no. 2 (June 2004): 287-301, www.learcenter.org/pdf/BBHotline.pdf (accessed November 30, 2008).

22  Karen Donelan, Peter Buerhaus, Catherine Desroches, Robert Dittus and David Dutwin, "Public Perceptions of Nursing Careers: The Influence of the Media and Nursing Shortages," Nursing Economics 26, no. 3 (2008), www.medscape.com/viewarticle/576950 (accessed December 2, 2008).

23  Dianne Felblinger, "Incivility and Bullying in the Workplace and Nurses' Shame Responses," Journal of Obstetric, Gynecologic, & Neonatal Nursing 37,

no. 2 (March/April 2008): 234-42, http://tinyurl.com/6s28ut (accessed November 30, 2008), summary available at http://healthnews.uc.edu/news /?/6716/.

## CHAPTER 3: Could Monkeys Be Nurses?

1 Daniel Simons and Christopher Chabris, "Gorillas In Our Midst: Sustained Inattentional Blindness for Dynamic Events," *Perception* 28 (1999): 1059-74, www.wjh.harvard.edu/~cfc/Simons1999.pdf; video available at http://viscog.beckman.uiuc.edu/grafs/demos/15.html (accessed May 25, 2008).

## CHAPTER 4: Yes, Doctor! No, Doctor!

1 California Nursing Practice Act, Business & Professions Code § 2725. See generally Cal. Bus. & Prof. Code §§ 2725-2742 (Nursing — Scope of Regulation), http://www.rn.ca.gov/regulations/bpc.shtml, http://tinyurl .com/6cn3gb (accessed December 2, 2008).

## CHAPTER 5: The Naughtiest Nurse

1 Tammy McGuire, Debbie Dougherty and Joshua Atkinson, "Paradoxing the Dialectic: The Impact of Patients' Sexual Harassment in the Discursive Construction of Nurses' Caregiving Roles," *Management Communication Quarterly* 19, no. 3 (2006): 416-50, http://mcq.sagepub.com/cgi/content/ abstract/19/3/416 (accessed July 20, 2008). See Mildred L. Culp, "Patients Harassing Nurses? Oh, Yes! How Nurses, Administrators and Society Can Respond," *Nursing in Virginia Magazine* (Spring 2006), www .nursinginva.com/spring2006/patients-harassing.htm (accessed July 19, 2008); John Rossheim, "How Nurses Can Fight Sexual Harassment," *Monster* (March 2006), http://content.monster.com/articles/3493/17214/1/ home.aspx (accessed November 30, 2008).

2 Tamra B. Orr, "Danger Zone," *NurseWeek,* November 4, 2002, www .nurseweek.com/news/features/02-11/dangerzone_web.asp (accessed July 20, 2008).

3 Associated Press, "Inappropriate Patient Behavior Tough on Nurses: Sexual Harassment a Widespread Problem, Health Officials Say," December 15, 2005, www.msnbc.msn.com/id/10484939/from/RL.2/ (accessed October 18, 2008).

4 P. Glick, S. Weber, C. Johnson and H. Branstiter, "Evaluations of Sexy Women in Low and High Status Jobs," *Psychology of Women Quarterly* 29, no. 4 (December 2005): 389-95, http://tinyurl.com/6nx7r8 (accessed

November 30, 2008). See Eric Noe, "Can Sexy Women Climb the Corporate Ladder? A New Study Suggests that Bold, Revealing Clothing May Keep You from Getting a Promotion," ABC News, December 2, 2005, http://abcnews.go.com/Business/Science/story?id=1362956 (accessed October 18, 2008).

## CHAPTER 6: Who Wants Yesterday's Girl?

1 Karen A. Hart, "Study: Who Are the Men in Nursing?" *Imprint* (November / December 2005): 32-34, www.nsna.org/pubs/imprint/novdec05/imp_nov05%20breakthough.pdf (accessed July 20, 2008).

2 JWT Communications, "Memo to Nurses for a Healthier Tomorrow Coalition Members on Focus Group Studies of 1,800 School Children in 10 U.S. Cities" (2000), www.nursingadvocay.org/research/lit/jwt_memo1.html.

3 Karen A. Hart, "Breakthrough to Nursing National Survey Results," *Imprint* (February / March 2006): 29-33, www.nsna.org/pubs/imprint/febmar05/ime20_columns_BTN.pdf (accessed November 30, 2008).

4 Joan Sosin, "Indecent Proposals: Nurses Experiencing Harassment, Discrimination in the Workplace Are Reminded that the Law Is on Their Side," *NurseWeek,* February 28, 2003, www.nurseweek.com/news/features/03-02/discrimination.asp (accessed July 15, 2008).

## CHAPTER 8: Winning the Battle-Axe, Losing the War

1 Linda S. Smith, "Image Counts: Greeting Cards Mail It in When It Comes to Accurately Portraying Nurses," *Nursing Spectrum*, Southern ed., October 1, 2003, www2.nursingspectrum.com/articles/print.html?AID=10528 (accessed November 28, 2008).

## CHAPTER 9:
## APRNs: Skilled Professionals or Cut-Rate "Physician Extenders"?

1 U.S. Department of Health and Human Services, "The Registered Nurse Population: Findings from the 2004 National Sample Survey of Registered Nurses: Chapter III: The Registered Nurse Population 2004" (2004), http://bhpr.hrsa.gov/healthworkforce/rnsurvey04/3.htm (accessed August 19, 2008).

2 American Academy of Nurse Practitioners, "Frequently Asked Questions," www.npfinder.com/faq.pdf (accessed July 29, 2008).

3 National Association of Clinical Nurse Specialists, "Frequently Asked Questions," www.nacns.org/faqs.shtml (accessed July 29, 2008).

4  U.S. Department of Health and Human Services, "The Registered Nurse Population: Findings from the 2004 National Sample Survey of Registered Nurses: Tables," http://bhpr.hrsa.gov/healthworkforce/rnsurvey04/appendixa.htm (accessed August 19, 2008).

5  Center for Nursing Advocacy, "Do Physicians Deliver Better Care than Advanced Practice Registered Nurses?" www.nursingadvocacy.org/faq/apn_md_relative_merits.html.

6  American Academy of Nurse Anesthetists, "Introduction to Quality of Care in Anesthesia," http://tinyurl.com/6ocgwr (accessed July 27, 2008).

7  Debra J. Jackson, Janet M. Lang, William H. Swartz, Theodore G. Ganiats, Judith Fullerton, Jeffrey Ecker and Uyensa Nguyen, "Outcomes, Safety, and Resource Utilization in a Collaborative Care Birth Center Program Compared with Traditional Physician-Based Perinatal Care," *American Journal of Public Health* 93, no. 6 (June 2003): 999-1006, www.ajph.org/cgi/content/full/93/6/999 (accessed August 19, 2008).

8  Sue Horrocks, Elizabeth Anderson and Chris Salisbury, "Systematic Review of Whether Nurse Practitioners Working in Primary Care Can Provide Equivalent Care to Doctors," *British Medical Journal* 324 (April 6, 2002): 819-23, www.bmj.com/cgi/content/full/324/7341/819 (accessed November 28, 2008).

9  M. O. Mundinger, R. L. Kane, E. R. Lenz, A. M. Totten, W. Y. Tsai, P. D. Cleary, W. T. Friedewald, A. L. Siu and M. L. Shelanski, "Primary Care Outcomes in Patients Treated by Nurse Practitioners or Physicians: A Randomized Trial," *Journal of the American Medical Association* 283, no. 1 (January 5, 2000): 59-68, www.ncbi.nlm.nih.gov/pubmed/10632281 (accessed October 18, 2008).

10  Sharon A. Brown and Deanna E. Grimes, "A Meta-Analysis of Nurse Practitioners and Nurse Midwives in Primary Care," *Nursing Research* 44, no. 6 (November/December 1995): 332-9, http://tinyurl.com/6q66ut (accessed November 28, 2008).

11  Center for Nursing Advocacy, "Nurses Are About 100 Times More Likely To Attend Graduate Nursing School than Medical School," www.nursingadvocacy.org/news/nursing_school_stats.html.

**CHAPTER 10:** How We Can All Improve Understanding of Nursing

1  Google, "Google Health Advisory Council" (2007), www.google.com/intl/en-US/health/about/ghac.html (accessed August 17, 2008).

2 Sion E. Rogers, "'Me and My Shadow' Is Mantra for a New Medical Student Elective," *Dartmouth Medicine Magazine* (Summer 2005), http://dartmed.dartmouth.edu/summer05/html/vs_mantra.php (accessed October 5, 2008).

**CHAPTER 11** How Nurses Can Improve Their Own Image

1 *Today Show*, "What Your Hospital Doesn't Want You to Know," NBC (September 21, 2006), http://tinyurl.com/4h9k25 (accessed November 30, 2008).

2 Sandy Summers, "The Nursing Uniform of Tomorrow: Transforming the Nursing Image from the Ground Up," available at www.nursingvision.org/uniforms.html.

3 Connecticut League for Nursing, "CLN to Host Nursing Leadership Conference" (March 23, 2005), www.ctleaguefornursing.org/pdf/press_032305.pdf (accessed August 16, 2008).

4 U.S. Department of Health and Human Services, Office for Civil Rights, "HIPAA Medical Privacy – National Standards to Protect the Privacy of Personal Health Information," www.hhs.gov/ocr/hipaa/ (accessed December 2, 2008). See also U.S. Department of Health and Human Services, Office of the Secretary, "Health Insurance Portability and Accountability Act of 1996, Public Law 104-191" (August 21, 1996), http://aspe.hhs.gov/admnsimp/pL104191.htm (accessed October 3, 2008).

5 California Nurses Association, "If He Were Anyone Else, He'd Probably Be Dead by Now" (print advertisement), *Washington Post* (May 2008), http://tinyurl.com/3a4ejr (accessed October 2, 2008).

6 Center for Nursing Advocacy, *ER* Action Center, www.nursingadvocacy.org/action/letters/er/er.html.

7 Institute for Healthcare Development, "Who's Using These Books?" www.iha4health.org/index.cfm/MenuItemID/210.htm (accessed October 7, 2008).

8 Health On the Net Foundation, "About Health On the Net Foundation," www.hon.ch/Global/HON_mission.html (accessed October 27, 2008).

**Information about nearly all materials discussed in this book that are not referenced in the endnotes can be found through the search engine on the Center for Nursing Advocacy's website at www.nursingadvocacy.org. If you cannot find information there, please contact info@nursingadvocacy.org.

# REFERENCES

## Action Center

Center for Nursing Advocacy, "What can you do to shape a better image of nursing? Take action with our plan to remedy the nursing image and the nursing profession," www.nursingadvocacy.org/action/action .html.

Buresh, Bernice, and Suzanne Gordon. 2006. *From Silence to Voice*, 2nd ed. Ithaca: Cornell University Press.

Center for Nursing Advocacy, "Chapters of the Center for Nursing Advocacy," www.nursingadvocacy.org/chapters/chapters.html.

Center for Nursing Advocacy, "*Grey's Anatomy* Action Page," www .nursingadvocacy.org/action/letters/2005/greys_anatomy/greys.html.

Center for Nursing Advocacy, "*House* Action Page," www.nursingadvocacy .org/action/letters/house/house.html.

Center for Nursing Advocacy, "*Private Practice* Action Page," www .nursingadvocacy.org/action/letters/2007/private_practice/pp.html.

Center for Nursing Advocacy, "*ER* Action Page," www.nursingadvocacy .org/action/letters/er/er.html.

Center for Nursing Advocacy, "*Scrubs* Action Page," www.nursingadvocacy .org/action/letters/scrubs/scrubs.html.

## The Media's Effect on Nursing

Center for Nursing Advocacy, "Q: Come on. Even if the mass media does ignore nursing, or present it inaccurately, how can that possibly affect nursing in real life?" www.nursingadvocacy.org/faq/media_affects_ nursing.html.

Center for Nursing Advocacy, "Q: OK, fine. I can see that some media probably affects how people think about and act toward nursing, like maybe a respected newspaper or current affairs show on TV. But how can some TV drama, sitcom or commercial affect people that way? People know enough not to take that stuff seriously!" www.nursingadvocacy.org/faq/media_affects_thinking.html.

Center for Nursing Advocacy, "Q: I get that the public health community and even Hollywood itself believes that the entertainment media has a big effect on real world health. But is there any actual research showing it affects what people think and do about health issues like nursing?" www.nursingadvocacy.org/faq/hollywood_research.html.

Center for Nursing Advocacy, "Q: Well, if all that research shows how influential Hollywood is on health care — and Hollywood itself claims credit for improving the world through medical accuracy — why won't it admit that its portrayal of nursing is equally influential, and take steps to fix it? Especially since the nursing shortage is now a global public health crisis," www.nursingadvocacy.org/faq/hollywood_behavior.html.

Center for Nursing Advocacy, "Q: Nurses are just wonderful, but you really can't expect Hollywood to focus on them, can you? After all, popular media products have to be dramatic and exciting. Why don't you just focus on getting a nursing documentary on PBS or basic cable?" www.nursingadvocacy.org/faq/dramatic.html.

Gordon, Suzanne. 2005. *Nursing Against the Odds: How Health Care Cost-Cutting, Media Stereotypes, and Medical Hubris Undermine Nursing and Patient Care.* Ithaca: Cornell University Press.

Buresh, Bernice, and Suzanne Gordon. 2006. *From Silence to Voice*, 2nd ed. Ithaca: Cornell University Press.

Kalisch, Beatrice, and Phillip Kalisch. "The Work of Beatrice Kalisch and Philip Kalisch on Nursing's Public Image and the Nursing Shortage," www.nursingadvocacy.org/research/lit/kalisch_kalisch.html.

Buresh, Bernice, Suzanne Gordon and Nica Bell. 1991. "Who Counts in News Coverage of Health Care?" *Nursing Outlook* 39, no. 5, (September/October): 204-208.

University of Rochester School of Nursing. 1997. "Woodhull Study on Nursing and the Media: Health Care's Invisible Partner," Sigma Theta Tau International, www.nursingsociety.org/Media/Pages/woodhall.aspx.

Glik, Deborah. 2003. Health Communication in Popular Media Formats. Paper presented at the 131st annual meeting of the American Public Health Association, November 15–19 in San Francisco, California, www.medscape.com/viewarticle/466709.

JWT Communications. 2000. "Memo to Nurses for a Healthier Tomorrow on a Focus Group Study of 1800 School Children in 10 US Cities," www.nursingadvocacy.org/research/lit/jwt_memo1.html.

Kaiser Family Foundation. 2004. "Entertainment Education and Health in the United States," www.kff.org/entmedia/7047.cfm.

Kaiser Family Foundation. 2008. "Hollywood & Health: Health Content in Entertainment Television," www.kff.org/entmedia/mho91608pkg.cfm

Kaiser Family Foundation. 2002. "The Impact of TV's Health Content: A Case Study of ER Viewers," www.kff.org/entmedia/3230-index.cfm.

Smith, Linda S. 2003. "Image Counts: Greeting Cards Mail It in When It Comes to Accurately Portraying Nurses." Nursing Spectrum, (Southern ed.), October 1, www2.nursingspectrum.com/articles/print.html?AID=10528.

Turow, Joseph, and Rachel Gans. 2002. "As Seen on TV: Health Policy Issues in TV's Medical Dramas," Report to the Kaiser Family Foundation, www.kff.org/entmedia/3231-index.cfm.

## Autonomy in Nursing

Center for Nursing Advocacy, "Q: Are You Sure Nurses Are Autonomous? Based On What I've Seen, It Sure Looks Like Physicians Are Calling the Shots," www.nursingadvocacy.org/faq/autonomy.html.

Center for Nursing Advocacy, "Review of Nursing Against the Odds," www.nursingadvocacy.org/media/books/nursing_against_odds.html.

## The Nursing Shortage

Center for Nursing Advocacy, "Q: What Is the Nursing Shortage and Why Does It Exist?" www.nursingadvocacy.org/faq/nursing_shortage .html.

Center for Nursing Advocacy, "Problems Thwarting Nursing Recruitment and Retention," www.nursingadvocacy.org/faq/recruit_retain.html.

Gordon, Suzanne. 2005. *Nursing against the Odds: How Health Care Cost-Cutting, Media Stereotypes, and Medical Hubris Undermine Nursing and Patient Care.* Ithaca: Cornell University Press.

International Council of Nurses. 2004. "The Global Shortage of Registered Nurses: An Overview of Issues and Actions," www.icn.ch/global/shortage.pdf.

American Association of Colleges of Nursing, "Nurse Reinvestment Act at a Glance," www.aacn.nche.edu/Media/NRAataglance.htm.

American Association of Colleges of Nursing, "Nursing Shortage Resource," www.aacn.nche.edu/media/shortageresource.htm.

U.S. Department of Labor, Bureau of Labor Statistics, "Registered Nurses," www.bls.gov/oco/ocos083.htm.

Buerhaus, Peter, Douglas Staiger and David Auerbach. 2008. *The Future of the Nursing Workforce in the United States: Data, Trends and Implications.* Boston: Jones and Bartlett Publishers, www.jbpub .com/catalog/9780763756840/.

### NURSE MIGRATION

Center for Nursing Advocacy, "Q: How is nurse migration affecting nurses and the nursing shortage?" www.nursingadvocacy.org/faq/migration .html.

Kingma, Mireille. 2006. *Nurses on the Move: Migration and the Global Health Care Economy.* Ithaca: Cornell University Press.

### MINIMUM NURSE-TO-PATIENT RATIOS

Center for Nursing Advocacy, "What happens to patients when nurses are short-staffed?" www.nursingadvocacy.org/faq/shortstaffed.html.

Gordon, Suzanne, John Buchanan and Tanya Bretherton. 2008. *Safety in Numbers*. Ithaca: Cornell University Press.

California Nurses Association, "RN-to-Patient Ratios," www.calnurses .org/nursing-practice/ratios/ratios_index.html.

Massachusetts Nurses Association, "Safe Care Campaign," www.massnurses .org/safe_care/index.htm.

Center for Nursing Advocacy, "Groundbreaking Study Shows that Nurse Short-Staffing Increases Patient Mortality, Nursing Dissatisfaction and Nursing Burnout," www.nursingadvocacy.org/news/2002oct23_jama .html.

Center for Nursing Advocacy, "No Magic Number," www.nursingadvocacy .org/news/2006/jan/21_abc.html.

Gordon, Suzanne. 2005. *Nursing Against the Odds: How Health Care Cost-Cutting, Media Stereotypes, and Medical Hubris Undermine Nursing and Patient Care*. Ithaca: Cornell University Press.

Weinberg, Dana Beth. 2003. *Code Green: Money-Driven Hospitals and the Dismantling of Nursing*. Ithaca: Cornell University Press.

## PHYSICIAN DISRUPTIVE BEHAVIOR

Center for Nursing Advocacy, "What is physician disruptive behavior and why does it exist?" www.nursingadvocacy.org/faq/disruptive_behavior .html.

Rosenstein, Alan H. 2002. "Nurse-Physician Relationships: Impact on Nurse Satisfaction and Retention." *American Journal of Nursing* 102, no. 6, (June): 26-34, www.nursingcenter.com/library/JournalArticle .asp?Article_ID=278949.

Mason, Diana J. 2002. "MD-RN: A Tired Old Dance." *American Journal of Nursing* 102, no. 6, (June): 7, www.nursingcenter.com/library/ JournalArticle.asp?Article_ID=278965.

University of Cincinnati. 2008. "Bullying Threatens Patient Care and Nurses' Careers," *Health News* (March 26), http://healthnews.uc.edu/ news/?/6716/.

## SEXUAL HARASSMENT

McGuire, Tammy, Debbie Dougherty and Joshua Atkinson. 2006. "Paradoxing the Dialectic: The Impact of Patients' Sexual Harassment in the Discursive Construction of Nurses' Caregiving Roles." *Management Communication Quarterly* 19:3, 416-50, http://mcq.sagepub.com/cgi/content/abstract/19/3/416.

Orr, Tamra. 2002. "Danger Zone." *NurseWeek*, November 4, www.nurseweek.com/news/features/02-11/dangerzone_web.asp.

Rossheim, John. 2006. "How Nurses Can Fight Sexual Harassment," *Monster*, (March) http://content.monster.com/articles/3493/17214/1/home.aspx.

Associated Press. 2005. "Inappropriate Patient Behavior Tough on Nurses: Sexual Harassment a Widespread Problem, Health Officials Say." December 15, www.msnbc.msn.com/id/10484939/from/RL.2/.

Noe, Eric. 2005. "Can Sexy Women Climb the Corporate Ladder? A New Study Suggests That Bold, Revealing Clothing May Keep You from Getting a Promotion." ABC News, December 2, http://abcnews.go.com/Business/Science/story?id=1362956.

Glick, Peter, Sadie Weber, Cathryn Johnson, and Heather Branstiter. 2005. "Evaluations of Sexy Women in Low- and High-Status Jobs." *Psychology of Women Quarterly* 29: 389-95, http://tinyurl.com/6a4kl3.

Sosin, Joan. 2003. "Indecent Proposals: Nurses Experiencing Harassment, Discrimination in the Workplace Are Reminded That the Law Is on Their Side." *NurseWeek*, February 28, www.nurseweek.com/news/features/03-02/discrimination.asp.

Culp, Mildred L. 2006. "Patients Harassing Nurses? Oh, Yes! How Nurses, Administrators and Society Can Respond," *Nursing in Virginia*, Spring, www.nursinginva.com/spring2006/patients-harassing.htm.

## NURSING EDUCATION LEVEL

Center for Nursing Advocacy, "Aiken Places another Major Study in *JAMA*, Linking Bachelor's-Prepared Nurses with Lower Patient Mortality; Much of Elite Media Yawns," www.nursingadvocacy.org/news/2003sep26_ap.html.

Center for Nursing Advocacy, "No Magic Number," www.nursingadvocacy
.org/news/2006/jan/21_abc.html.

TRAVEL NURSING

Center for Nursing Advocacy, "Would You Like a Krabby Patty with
That?" www.nursingadvocacy.org/news/2006/mar/17_balt_sun.html.

## Nursing Faculty Shortage

Nurses for a Healthier Tomorrow, "Careers in Nursing Campaign,"
www.nursesource.org/campaign_newsCIN.html.

American Association of Colleges of Nurses, "Nursing Faculty
Shortage Fact Sheet," www.aacn.nche.edu/media/backgrounders/
facultyshortage.htm.

National League for Nursing. 2007. "Key Findings of Nationwide
NLN–Carnegie Foundation: Study of Nurse Educators Released,"
www.nln.org/newsreleases/carnegie_082907.htm.

## Advanced Practice Nurses

Center for Nursing Advocacy, "Do Physicians Deliver Better Care than
Advanced Practice Registered Nurses?" www.nursingadvocacy.org/
faq/apn_md_relative_merits.html.

American Academy of Nurse Anesthetists, "Introduction to Quality of
Care in Anesthesia," http://tinyurl.com/6ocgwr.

## Who Are APRNs and What Do They Do?

American Academy of Nurse Practitioners. "Frequently Asked Questions," www.npfinder.com/faq.pdf.

National Association of Clinical Nurse Specialists. "Frequently Asked
Questions," www.nacns.org/faqs.shtml.

## Angel Stereotype

Center for Nursing Advocacy, "Are Nurses Angels of Mercy?" www
.nursingadvocacy.org/faq/nf/are_nurses_angels.html.

Center for Nursing Advocacy, "Q: Don't You Want Nurses To Be Compassionate? You Seem Uncomfortable When Nurses Are Described That Way, And You Focus Instead on Nurses' Training and Skills," www.nursingadvocacy.org/faq/compassion.html.

Center for Nursing Advocacy, "Touching the World," www.nursing-advocacy.org/media/commercials/jnj_2005.html.

Center for Nursing Advocacy, "Male Nurse Action Figures and the Pink Pearlized Heart Shaped Messages of Faith and Love," www.nursingadvocacy.org/news/2004oct/angels.html.

Gordon, Suzanne. 2005. *Nursing Against the Odds: How Health Care Cost-Cutting, Media Stereotypes, and Medical Hubris Undermine Nursing and Patient Care.* Ithaca: Cornell University Press.

Buresh, Bernice, and Suzanne Gordon. 2006. *From Silence to Voice*, 2nd ed. Ithaca: Cornell University Press.

## Naughty Nurse Stereotype

Center for Nursing Advocacy, "Q: What's the Big Deal About Naughty Nurse Images In the Media? I Mean, No One Believes Nurses Really Dress Like That!" www.nursingadvocacy.org/faq/naughty_nurse.html.

Center for Nursing Advocacy, "Q: But I'm Young And Hot and I Love People To Think Nurses Are Sexy! Promiscuous Girls Rule! Anyone Who Objects To the Naughty Nurse Image Must Be an Old Hag Nursing Leader Who Hates Sex and Freedom, Right?" www.nursingadvocacy.org/faq/hotness.html.

## Magnet Status

Center for Nursing Advocacy, "What Is Magnet Status and How's That Whole Thing Going?" www.nursingadvocacy.org/faq/magnet.html.

## Good Media on Nursing

*Nursing Diaries: Part One: The Rookies.* 2004. Directed by Richard Kahn and Linda Martin, information available at www.nursingadvocacy.org/media/documentaries/nursing_diaries.html.

Rap Recruiting Video. 2004. Created by Craig Barton, information available at www.nursingadvocacy.org/media/recruitment/barton_rap.html.

*Angels in America.* 2003. Directed by Tony Kushner, information available at www.nursingadvocacy.org/media/films/angels.html.

"Critical Care: The Making of an ICU Nurse." 2005. Written by Scott Allen, photographs by Michele McDonald, *The Boston Globe*, October 23–26, information available at www.nursingadvocacy.org/news/2005oct/23_boston_globe.html.

"Swamp Nurse." 2006. Katherine Boo, *The New Yorker*, February 6, information available at www.nursingadvocacy.org/news/2006/feb/06_swamp_nurse.html.

*Nurses.* 2002. A five-part documentary series by Helen Holt, information available at www.nursingadvocacy.org/media/documentaries/nurses.html.

*Wit.* 2001. Directed by Mike Nichols; screenplay by Emma Thompson and Mike Nichols, information available at www.nursingadvocacy.org/media/films/wit.html.

Male Nurse Action Figure, Archie McPhee, information available at www.nursingadvocacy.org/news/2004oct/angels.html#mcphee.

## Men in Nursing

Center for Nursing Advocacy, "Yo, Dog, What's Up with this Nursing Thing? Are You Nuts?" www.nursingadvocacy.org/faq/men_in_nursing.html.

JWT Communications. 2000. "Memo to Nurses for a Healthier Tomorrow Coalition Members on Focus Group Studies of 1,800 School Children in 10 U.S. Cities," www.nursingadvocay.org/research/lit/jwt_memo1.html.

Hart, Karen. 2005. "Study: Who Are the Men in Nursing?" Bernard Hodes Group, www.nsna.org/pubs/imprint/novdec05/imp_novo5%20breakthough.pdf. See also Karen A. Hart. 2005. "Men in Nursing Survey: First of its Kind Survey of Male Nurses." *Imprint*, (November/December 2005): 32–34, www.nsna.org/pubs/imprint/febmar05/ime20_columns_BTN.pdf.

Center for Nursing Advocacy, "Problems Thwarting Nursing Recruitment and Retention," www.nursingadvocacy.org/faq/recruit_retain.html.

## Educating Physicians

Sion E. Rogers, "'Me and My Shadow' Is Mantra for a New Medical Student Elective," *Dartmouth Medicine Magazine* (Summer 2005), http://dartmed.dartmouth.edu/summer05/html/vs_mantra.php.

## Nursing Uniforms

Sandy Summers, "The Nursing Uniform of Tomorrow: Transforming the Nursing Image from the Ground Up," www.nursingvision.org/uniforms.html.

Center for Nursing Advocacy, "Wear the RN Patch! Join us in creating a professional nursing uniform," www.nursingadvocacy.org/action/RN_patch.html.

# INDEX

# ABOUT THE CENTER
# FOR NURSING ADVOCACY

REGISTERED NURSES ARE the critical front-line caregivers in health care today. For millions of people worldwide, nurses are the difference between life and death, self-sufficiency and dependency, hope and despair. Yet a lack of true appreciation for nursing has led to a shortage that is one of our most urgent public health crises. The nursing shortage has claimed countless lives and is overwhelming the world's health systems. It is no exaggeration to say that the future depends on a better understanding of nursing.

The Center for Nursing Advocacy is an international non-profit organization working to meet that challenge. It was founded by a group of seven graduate students at Johns Hopkins University School of Nursing in 2001. The Center tells the media and the public what nurses really do. It analyzes the media's treatment of nurses, helping nurses stand together to end harmful depictions and encourage accurate ones. Better public understanding of nursing will lead to more social, political, and financial support for the profession, which will in turn relieve the nursing shortage and improve the health of all people.

Visit the Center at www.nursingadvocacy.org.

All royalties from this book go to support the Center for Nursing Advocacy. However, the views expressed in the book are those of the authors, and do not necessarily reflect the views of the Center for Nursing Advocacy.

# ABOUT THE AUTHORS

SANDY SUMMERS has served as executive director of the Center for Nursing Advocacy since 2001, when she founded the organization with other graduate nursing students at Johns Hopkins University. She frequently speaks to the media and at conferences. In 2002 Summers earned master's degrees in community health nursing and public health from Johns Hopkins. She also has a BSN degree from Southern Connecticut State University. Prior to her graduate work, Summers practiced nursing for fifteen years in the emergency departments and intensive care units of major U.S. trauma centers, including public hospitals in San Francisco, New Orleans, and Washington, DC. In the mid-1990s, she worked in Phnom Penh, Cambodia, where she taught nursing teachers at the Central Nursing School. And she practiced ICU nursing for a year at a hospital on St. Thomas in the U.S. Virgin Islands.

HARRY JACOBS SUMMERS has been senior adviser to the Center for Nursing Advocacy since 2003, also serving as the group's main writer. He has an undergraduate degree from Columbia University and a law degree from Georgetown University. Summers studied for a year on a Fulbright scholarship in New Zealand. He also taught and provided advice on commercial law to government officials in Phnom Penh, Cambodia, for three years. Since 1998 he has been a litigation attorney at the Federal Election Commission, which enforces federal election campaign law, in Washington, DC.

Sandy and Harry have co-authored articles on nursing and the media for major nursing journals and textbooks. They live in Baltimore with their two children.

The authors can be contacted at authors@savinglivesthebook.org.